ALONE IN THE WORLD

Alone in the World

STORIES OF COMPLEX HUMAN RELATIONSHIPS

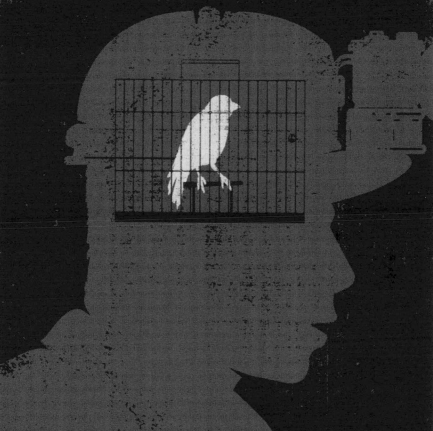

Ashok Kumar, MD.

ISBN-13:9780692551950
ISBN-10: 0692551956

To my parents and my patients—my greatest teachers

TABLE OF CONTENTS

ACKNOWLEDGMENTS

Thank you to my staff for the love, caring, and dedication that you have shown to our patients and me. Thank you for the thousands of afternoon cups of coffee over the past thirty years and the sincerity that went into them.

A special acknowledgement to Christine Retz, my editor and my friend. You have been a valuable guide through this journey. Thank you for fine-tuning my words so that my stories could be better heard.

Finally, I would like to thank my children and my wife, Vijay, for their love and support, and constantly encouraging me to take on the next endeavor.

A man is defined by the lifestyle and rituals that he follows, not the god he worships. Prayer is an integral part of the Hindu tradition. No journey is undertaken without this ritual. Writing this book was a monumental task—a long trip. In keeping with Hindu rituals, I would like to share with you a prayer given to me as a gift from a person in religious life.

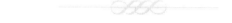

DAILY PRAYER OF THE PHYSICIAN

Almighty God, you have created the human body with infinite wisdom. In your eternal providence, you have chosen me to watch over the life and health of your creatures. I am now about to apply myself to the duties of my profession. Support me in these great labors that they may benefit humankind, for without your help, not even the least thing will succeed.

Inspire me with love for my art and for your creatures. Do not allow thirst for profit or ambition for renown and admiration to interfere with my profession, for these are the enemies of truth and can lead me astray in the great task of attending to the welfare of your creatures. Preserve the strength of my body and soul that they may ever be ready to help rich and poor, good and bad, and enemy and friend. In the sufferer let me see only the human being.

Enlighten my mind that it may recognize what presents itself and that it may comprehend what is absent or hidden. Let it not fail to see what is visible, but do not permit it to arrogate to itself the power to see what cannot be seen, for delicate and indefinite are the bounds of the great art of caring for the lives and health of your creatures. May no strange thoughts divert my attention at the bedside of the sick or disturb my mind in its silent labors.

Grant that my patients may have confidence in me and my art and follow my directions and my counsel. When those who are wiser than me wish to instruct me, let my soul gratefully follow their guidance, for vast is the extent of our art. Imbue my soul with gentleness and calmness. Let me be contented in everything except in the great science of my profession. Never allow the thought to arise in me that I have attained sufficient knowledge, but grant me the strength and ambition to extend my knowledge. The art is great, but the mind of a person is ever expanding. I now rise to my calling.

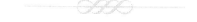

INTRODUCTION

This book is a series of case studies that examine how illness affects our lives as human beings, and how disease affects our relationships, our marriages, and our entire world. Patients struggle to deal with sickness and the many issues that come along with any given diagnosis. Sometimes, for example, a man is less concerned with his illness and more worried about his status as husband and father. At times, after a debilitating illness like a heart attack or a stroke, a patient's social landscape changes, and the people he or she was counting on move on with their lives. A spouse can become an impediment to recovery or the cure. In some cases, the relationship between husband and wife strengthens. In other cases, the love between husband and wife vanishes like the morning dew. It could be that relationships patients build all their lives turn out to be illusions.

It is these nonmedical consequences of disease that are the hardest for patients to deal with—and are often ignored by the doctor. We doctors have mastered the art of treating medical pathology; however, we practically ignore the human condition.

In my practice, I follow a set ritual. First, I examine the patient, and then I examine his or her social infrastructure. The former is often easier to address than the latter. Over the past twenty-eight years, I have found that it is easy to put a stent in the heart. However, to mend a broken heart, the patient will need more than pills and complicated procedures.

We start the office visit with a physical examination. Then I invite both the patient and his or her family to join me in my consultation room. Most of my time is devoted to evaluating the dynamics of their relationship and how the illness has impacted them.

As a young doctor, I spent the majority of my time in the examination room. That was when I practiced medicine and focused only on treating disease. As I evolved as a physician, I came to realize that the true healing was happening in the consultation room where I could help patients and families restore some balance. The right social support is paramount to a patient's recovery, and as a doctor, I feel it is my duty to advocate that for my patients.

The following case studies reflect my time in the consultation room with my patients—the place where I believe the real healing occurs.

Nothing is more powerful than an
idea whose time has come.

—Victor Hugo

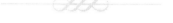

AN ATHEIST

No atheists have killed people in the name of their ideology or philosophy.

Pete, a sixty-five-year-old retired teacher, came to the office for an evaluation of chest pain. His present illness started a month ago. While walking briskly to catch the train to New York City, he experienced retrosternal chest pressure accompanied by shortness of breath. He had no complaint of palpitation or cold sweats, but he'd had a dizzy spell and felt weak during the chest pain. There was no history of radiation of chest pain to the left arm. He did not pay much attention to it because the pain subsided after resting for a while.

When I probed further, he told me that last month while canoeing in a lake he'd had a similar episode of chest pain. This time, the chest pain was severe, crushing, and debilitating. He decided to see his primary care physician, who referred him to me for further evaluation.

He had multiple risk factors for coronary artery disease,[1] including an abdominal aortic aneurysm[2] measuring about 4 cm in size, hypertension, and high cholesterol.

He drank Irish whiskey, but it was more than social drinking. He smoked one pack of cigarettes a day. His father died from a heart attack at age seventy.

"An atheist" was how he highlighted his faith with a red marker on the demographic sheet.

On physical examination, his features showed the effect of heavy drinking. It is well known that excessive drinking can take a toll on one's physical appearance. Pete had a slightly bloated face and reddened complexion. He had a gentle, friendly smile and straight hair parted in the middle. His blood pressure was normal; he had bilateral carotid bruits.[3] The chest examination revealed normal breath sounds, no rhonchcrep or crepitation,[4] and no signs of emphysema.[5] The cardiovascular examination showed a prominent S4 gallop[6] and an ejection systolic murmur[7] grade 2/6 in the aortic area. The abdominal and central nervous system were essentially unremarkable. The extremities' examination showed no sign of peripheral vascular disease,[8] and the EKG showed regular rhythm and no sign of a heart attack.

After the examination, I asked him to come to the consultation room.

"What is wrong?" he asked.

"You are suffering from unstable angina[9]—a step away from a heart attack. The best treatment option is an urgent admission to the hospital for further evaluation," I replied.

He politely declined my recommendation and wanted to be treated as an outpatient.

Pete's response to my warning surprised me. He must not have grasped the seriousness of his illness because a normal, thinking person would do everything in his or her power to prevent a heart attack.

"I have an important meeting to conduct," he explained.

"What kind of meeting?" I inquired.

"A humanist/atheist society meeting. It's important because there are forces working to undermine and hijack our goals, which are to build a prophetless religion that teaches gospel goodness without God." He elegantly articulated his faith, which is no faith.

His comments about building a "Godless" society startled me, and for a moment my thoughts went back to India and its diverse religious landscape. Growing up in India, I'd never met an atheist and had not taken care of an atheist as a patient. A large gap in religious orientation existed between me and Pete. I promised myself that I would follow my covenant as a physician and would not let this divide hinder my clinical judgment. The theology of atheism was as alien to me as the topography of a strange planet in the universe. India is a secular and spiritual country where there are countless temples, mosques, and churches coexisting in harmony. The life of a Hindu revolves around his or her God; the husband and wife both being Hindu can follow different deities. No religious hierarchy is micromanaging their relationship with God. In southern India, most Hindus start and end the day with prayer rituals. Nobody complains or gets mad if the bus driver decides to detour the bus to a temple to pray before starting a perilous journey.

In India, Shia and Sunni Muslims celebrate their rituals and festivals peacefully without the fear of getting hurt. They live in harmony. Islam has 1.7 million adherents (Sunni 85–86%, Shia 12–13%, and Ahmadis 1%). According to a 2010 Pew Research Center report, around 62% of the world's Muslims live in South and Southeast Asia, with over 1 billion followers. The study found more Muslims live in the United Kingdom than in Lebanon and more in China than in Syria. About 20% of Muslims live in the Arab countries.

According to the journalist Mustafa Akyol in a *New York Times* Op-Ed piece published on December 21, 2015, the right term to explain the theology of secular Islam is "irja." The word's literal meaning is "postponing." It was a theological principle put forward by some Muslim scholars during the first century of Islam. At that time the Muslim world was going through a major civil war. "The proponents of irja said that the burning question of who is a true Muslim should be 'postponed' until the afterlife. . . . Faith was a matter of the heart, something only God—not other human beings—could evaluate. The scholars who believed in the concept of irja were known as 'mirjia' or simply 'postponers.'"

When Islam arrived in India and Southeast Asia, Hinduism and Buddhism were the primary religions—teaching their adherents Vedanta and calming their minds through medita-tion. Islam and its teachings of love, compassion, and personal spiritual evolution were in harmony with the philosophy of local established religions. The symphony of diverse religions created a loving, all-inclusive society in India and Southeast

Asia. The Charaka Samhita and Sushruta Samhita – early texts on Ayurveda (Hindu traditional medicine) were translated in to Persian and Arabic by Hindu physicians working in the kingdoms of Muslim kings.

A Javanese mystical poem says:

"Many who memorize the Quran and Hadith love to condemn others as infidels, while ignoring their own infidelity to God, their hearts and minds still mired in filth."

The Muslims of India understand and practice true *jihad*—a personal spiritual evolution. Let God be the judge. In India, it is not uncommon to see Hindus praying at the tombs of Sufi (Muslim) saints.

A humble Catholic nun by the sheer strength of her faith in humanism, kindness, and altruism becomes a saint. To celebrate her kindness and humanism, in tradition-bound and spiritual India, Mother Teresa was given a state funeral, which is usually reserved for presidents and prime ministers.

In India, Christianity was established before some European nations had been Christianized, according to *Christianity in India* by Robert Eric Frykenberg. India ranks fifteenth among the countries with the highest church attendance. Good Friday is a national holiday. In areas such as Kerala (a state in southwestern India), where Christianity existed in pre-European times, land to build churches was donated by Hindu kings and Hindu landlords.

Judaism was one of the first foreign religions to arrive in India. Unlike other parts of the world, the Jews lived in India without any instances of anti-Semitism from the local Hindu-majority populace.

The Hindu king of Cochin permitted the Jews to live freely, to build synagogues, and to own properties "without conditions attached." The Mattancherry synagogue is the oldest active synagogue in Cochin—a port city in Kerala. It was built in 1567 by the Sephardic (Spanish) Jews. The land to build the synagogue was given to the Jews by the king. The Mattancherry Palace Hindu temple and Mattancherry synagogue share a common wall—polytheistic and monotheistic faiths coexisting in harmony—exploring the mysteries of the Vedas and Torah.

I grew up in spiritual India, where God is everywhere and very much alive. I think the strength of India's spirituality is its secular philosophy of tolerance and acceptance of religious diversity. Hinduism's historical tendency has been to recognize the divine basis of various religions, and to revere their founders and saintly practitioners. This continues today.

"What about God? What is wrong in having faith, to give meaning and purpose to life?" I asked.

Pete replied, "I have seen no reason to believe that any religion on Earth is anything more than man-made. As far as I am concerned, religion is a public show I never attend. This God, I'd like to meet him, but I don't want to take an organized trip. We should stop running after a father who has absconded to heaven and is never coming back (from *The Meursault Investigation*). I believe in a higher power, but not the kind of power proclaimed by most religions. I believe in God but not the Hindu, Muslim, or Christian God. I believe in Spinoza's God."

He continued, "I am not the only one who believes in Spinoza's God. Albert Einstein, John Dewey, and close to a billion people around the world believe in Spinoza's God."

"Do you think Baruch Spinoza or Albert Einstein were atheists?" I asked.

"Yes, they did not believe in a 'Jewish God,'" he replied.

I was not surprised to hear him say "Jewish God" instead of "God."

He continued, "Baruch Spinoza, born Benedito de Espinoza [November 24, 1632–February 21, 1677], was a Dutch Jewish philosopher. Spinoza's given name varies between different languages: in Hebrew it's Baruch Spinoza, in Portuguese Benedito de Espinoza, and in Latin Benedictus de Spinoza. In all these languages the given name means "Blessed." Spinoza was raised in the Portuguese Jewish community in Amsterdam. He was one of the most important and original thinkers of the seventeenth century. He had a vision of truth beyond what is granted to human beings. During Spinoza's life, the new science about the cosmos and the law of nature began to emerge. Armed with this knowledge, he started questioning the authenticity of the Hebrew Bible (the Tanakh) and dogma of Orthodox Judaism. Spinoza believed in God but not the traditional Jewish God. He redefined God as nature and as the universe itself. He saw God in the cosmos. He saw God's manifestations in Humanism and the kindness of Jewish people.

"Spinoza believed that we should interpret scripture on its own terms; interpretation of scripture by religious authorities is clouded by their motives to maintain power over people through ignorance.

"His thought on the philosophy of religion is best summarized in one of his famous quotes: 'Those who wish to seek out the cause of miracles and to understand the things of nature as philosophers, and not to stare at them in astonishment like fools, are soon considered heretical and impious and proclaimed as such by those whom the mob adores as the interpreters of nature and the God. These men know that once ignorance is put aside, that wonderment would be taken away, which is the only means by which their authority is preserved.'

"Spinoza argued that the stability and the security of society are enhanced by freedom of thought—the freedom to philosophize. His solution to religious orthodoxy was to strip clergy of all political and religious powers and give people freedom to interpret the nature of God. Spinoza's unorthodox views about religion and God strained his relationship with the synagogue. In 1656, he was excommunicated from the Jewish community. The elders burdened him with a reputation as an atheist— something he resented all his life.

"Spinoza was a Jew at the core of his consciousness and wanted to live a traditional Jewish life. He was not an atheist— he did not find God in rituals but found God in the cosmos and in nature.

"When someone asked Einstein if he believed in God, he responded, 'I believe in Spinoza's God who reveals himself in the harmony of nature.'

"In summary, for Baruch Spinoza and Albert Einstein, God was *'a question, not an answer,'*" Pete said with a mysterious smile. He continued, "The flame of pragmatism that was started by Baruch Spinoza will be kept burning, through many of his followers.

"Spinoza, a true pragmatist, inspired the American philosopher John Dewey [October 20, 1859–June 1, 1952]. The overriding theme of John Dewey's work was his profound belief in democracy and science. He believed that most philosophical topics, such as religious beliefs, are best viewed in terms of their practical uses and successes.

"He was a devout Christian. In his lecture entitled, 'The Obligation to Knowledge of God,' he emphasized the power of faith, not blind faith, but faith with knowledge. He said, 'Belief is not a privilege but a duty. Whatsoever is not of faith is sin.' In this lecture, he preached Hegel's philosophy of religion—"The Bible and Christianity should teach that humanity's highest duty is not only to love God but to know God.""

G. W. F. Hegel [August 27, 1770–November 14, 1831] was, by the time of his death, the most prominent philosopher in Germany. He was a rationalist and a moralist. The Gospel of Jesus, he said, is nothing if not a teaching of morals and ethics. Authoritarianism devalues free will and so devalues ethics. From Hegel's point of view, "an authoritarian religion is no religion."

The Hegelian dialectic—the idea that the truth is attained by synthesizing an idea (thesis) and its opposite (antithesis)—states that the two opposites are integrated and united to form a new concept (synthesis). Hegel applied this dialectic to study religion because, after all, "religion was a thesis—a man-made thesis."

After he died, Hegel's followers divided into right-wing and left-wing Hegelians. Theologically, the right-wing Hegelians offered a conservative interpretation of his work. They emphasized the compatibility between Hegel's philosophy and Christianity. The left-wing Hegelians interpreted his work as a validation of their belief in atheism. Karl Marx, the father of communism, was a left-wing Hegelian.

Pete's next comment surprised me. He said, "Pope Francis is a right-wing Hegelian because by welcoming gays and lesbians as God's children, he is making the Church less authoritarian."

He continued, "There is not much difference between Christianity and humanism/socialism—both preach altruism. Dewey said, 'God collects your sacrifices in one, society in the other.'

"In other words, by serving humanity, we are serving God. The rituals to please God will vary depending on the religion, but acts of altruism are the same whether you are Christian, Muslim, Jewish, or Hindu. All these roads (religions) are designed to take humankind to its final destination—to know God through his creation—through altruism and humanism.

There is a historical link—an unbroken chain of philosophical thoughts between Spinoza and the Indian secular constitution. Dewey's work and ideas about democracy and religion influenced one of his students, B. R. Ambedkar, who was the principal architect of the Indian Constitution. He strongly believed in secularism and science and wrote that 'the sovereignty of scriptures of all religions must come to an end if we want to have a united India.' Ambedkar was born to Hindu parents but did not like the way orthodox Hindus discriminated against the Untouchables, so he converted to Buddhism. Unlike Spinoza he was not excommunicated. The Hindu religion gave him space and freedom to find and know his God. He was appointed independent India's first minister of law.

He summarized his faith by saying, "Serving humanity and protecting the dignity of the poor and disadvantaged among us is more than enough reason to be kind and good without God. Nobody remembers or worships Roman gods, such as Janus (god of beginnings), Jupiter (king of the gods), Bellona (goddess of war), or Juno (queen of the gods). Man-made gods will come and go, and who knows how long our modern gods will be worshiped?"

In a strange way, I was happy that he was educating me about atheism. When he noticed that I was enjoying this conversation, he continued, "Atheists love India; it is where atheism started. Hinduism is the oldest religion in the world, and as we know, God and religion go hand in hand. Since the concept of religion and God started in India, obviously there were some members of the Hindu tribe who must have questioned and ridiculed the concept. In every society, there are believers as well as doubters. If the religion is ancient, so are humanism and atheism. The Rig Veda, a thirty-five-hundred-year-old collection of Sanskrit religious hymns, acknowledges and deals with atheism."

The Vedas are the most ancient religious texts that define truth for Hindus. Some Hindus believe that the texts were received by scholars directly from God and passed on to succeeding generations by word of mouth.

The Rig Veda is one of four Vedas, consisting of 1,028 religious hymns. It is the oldest Veda and deals with much skepticism regarding the fundamental question of our Creator God and the creation of the universe. In many instances, it does not categorically accept the existence of a Creator God. Nasadiya Sukta (a creation hymn) in the tenth chapter of Rig Veda states the following:

When was it produced? Whence is this creation?
The gods came afterward, with the creation of the universe.

HINDUISM IS A RELIGION BUT ALSO A PHILOSOPHY.

Madhava Acharya, a fourteenth-century philosopher, wrote a great book called *Sarva-Darsana-Samgraha*, which discusses all religious schools of thought within Hindu scripture. The first chapter discusses atheism—a very strong presentation of arguments in favor of atheism and materialism.

According to Markandey Katju, a former judge of the Supreme Court of India, there are six classical systems of Hindu philosophy: Nyaya, Vaisheshika, Sanka, Yoga, Purva Mimamsa, and Uttara Mimamsa. There are also three nonclassical systems: Buddhism, Jainism, and Charvaka (the ancient school of Indian materialism). Charvaka holds direct perception, empiricism, and conditional inference as proper sources of knowledge; embraces philosophical skepticism; and rejects Vedas, Vedic ritualism, and supernaturalism. Of these nine systems, eight of them are atheistic as there is no place for Creator God. Only the ninth one, Uttara Mimamsa, which is also called Vedanta, has a place for God in it as taught by Katju.

A word of advice to my non-Hindu friends and patients: by practicing yoga, you are following one of the classical Hindu philosophies, not the Hindu religion.

Yoga (from Sanskrit meaning "listen") is a physical, mental, and spiritual philosophy. It teaches us to listen to our inner core and reflect on life's blessings. It is one of the systems of classical Hindu philosophy.

Alexander the Great reached India in the fourth century BCE. Along with his army, he took Greek academics with him. One of Alexander's companions was Onesicritus. He described for the first time the yogis of India, who practiced aloofness and different postures to the Western world.

Onesicritus mentions that initially the yogis refused to meet him and his colleague Calanus, but later agreed because they were representing a "king curious for wisdom and philosophy."

Yoga's spiritual philosophy of life is to "rid the spirit of not only pain but pleasure. There is no shame in living on frugal fare. Live with undisturbed calmness and mindfulness through balance." Pope Francis embraces this concept, too.

Most people's knowledge of Hinduism stops at the popular perception that it has multiple gods. Hinduism has numerous prayers and rituals to please different gods, but it also has many schools of ancient philosophies, questioning and debating the basic concept of Creator God. Hinduism, a combination of religion and philosophy, deals with orthodoxy as well as atheism.

In an interview for the magazine *California* published in July–August 2006, the Indian Nobel Prize winner in Economics,

Amartya Sen, stated, "Sanskrit has a larger atheistic literature than what exists in any other classical language."

Hindu atheists accept Hinduism more as a way of life than religion.

Pete surprised me the most when he explained the origin of monotheistic philosophy by quoting Michel Onfray: "The lands of Israel, Judea, and Samaria of Jerusalem are desert, where the sun bakes men's heads and dehydrates their bodies and weakens their souls. The men who were exhausted and wandering in the unforgiving desert were yearning for oasis where water flows cool, clear, and free, and food is abundant. Heaven and the afterlife—the counterworld—is invented by these men. Monotheism was born of the sand."

He continued to discuss the fate of Christianity in America. Christianity is in decline because our culture is shifting. We are heading for a war—a cultural war between orthodox Christians and their positions on burning social issues like homosexuality, contraception, premarital sex, and mainstream culture—preaching the doctrine of humanism and inclusiveness. The Supreme Court's recent gay marriage decision was a body blow to the core of Christianity. This controversial decision will turbocharge the cultural balkanization of our society.

I was impressed by Pete's analysis. By the end of the appointment, I was able to appreciate his views about religion and God.

Before leaving the office, he encapsulated his faith in atheism by reciting Rabbi Sherwin Theodore Wine's poem, "Where Is My Light?" (Song of Humanistic Judaism):

Where is my light?
My light is in me.

Where is my hope?
My hope is in me.
Where is my strength?
My strength is in me—and in you.

Doctors who adopt a paternalistic approach are unlikely to learn from their patients. A shared approach to a patient's care is critical for a doctor's evolution as a healer.

Every patient has something to teach or to share, but unfortunately, we doctors waste a lot of time collecting useless data and staying ignorant about our patients' faith, fears, expectations, and disappointments. Our indifference toward nonmedical issues makes patients hesitant to share their beliefs and feelings; the fear of being ridiculed compels them to keep their inner thoughts—their psyches—hidden and protected.

Taking care of a patient without understanding and exploring his or her inner core is a job but half done.

I gave Pete enough time to explain his atheist philosophy, and I must confess that he educated and enlightened me about atheism. After meeting him, my biased views about atheism radically changed.

Pete was on a mission to save atheism from the forces of religious orthodoxy, and my job was to prevent his heart attack. In spite of my insistence, he refused to go to the hospital. His faith and commitment to atheism appeared to be unshakable. He was willing to sacrifice his health. I was impressed, and deep down in my heart, I liked him—he was a man of faith. I agreed to his request not to admit him in the hospital, and in return, he promised to come back for further testing. I had no choice but to bargain so that I could keep him under my care. I was hoping that he would come out a winner and not drop dead while debating the merits of atheism. He was advised to stop hunting and canoeing for the time being and take the medications I prescribed.

Humanists, atheists, priests, and rabbis are not in the business of absolute certainties. It is hard to prove that God does or does not exist, but I—being a cardiologist—was dealing with hard clinical facts. Pete's medical history was typical, indicating serious and life-threatening heart disease. I hated the fact that one of my patients was walking around with a time bomb ticking in his chest. I wanted to study him without wasting too much time; however, I had no choice but to wait for him to come back after saving atheism.

Before leaving the office, Pete signed all the necessary documents needed to proceed with cardiac testing. He was a member of a very prominent HMO that is intent on shackling health-care expenses to maximize profit by delaying or denying patients their needed care. For the patients who need urgent treatment, this is an adversarial system. The HMO will delay as a tactic of denial because most patients cannot sue their HMO for denial or delay of treatment and receive damages. The HMO has an incentive to stonewall, but sick patients may not have the time or energy for a struggle. Doctors taking care of these patients have to act on their behalf and negotiate with the HMO. Fighting with HMOs is like fighting with dinosaurs. They have all the legal and financial power to make decisions. No country in the world spends as much on health care as the United States or gets as little for its money. Much of this spending does not go into treatment. About one out of eight dollars spent by the health insurance companies goes into administrative costs, including lavish compensation for executives. As reported by the Health Administration Responsibility Project in 1996, the total annual compensation for the twenty-five highest-paid executives was $154 million, and total unexercised stock options valued $334.7 million. We spend nearly ten times what it costs the Canadian nationalized system.

The foundation and evolution of an inclusive, peaceful society is nurtured by the three most important fundamental human rights: food, shelter, and universal health.

I think HMOs are the ugliest face of merciless capitalism. No other civilized society will allow or tolerate this kind of health-care system in which the HMOs are empowered to play Russian roulette with people's health. The HMO is the classic example of how *privilege blinds*.

"We needed a prior authorization before booking Pete for a cardiac catheterization."[10] My nurse gave me this dreaded news.

After one week, the HMO denied my request to do a cardiac catheterization, stating, "The history of chest pain is insufficient information to give permission for the test." After sending multiple request forms and waiting, I finally got permission to do the cardiac catheterization.

Pete was admitted for cardiac catheterization. The test showed that he was suffering from subtotal stenosis[11] of the left main coronary artery (LMCA). About the size of the average cigarette butt, the LMCA is the most valuable section of the coronary arterial system within the body, and at least 75 percent of blood flow to the left ventricle is through this vessel. Studies performed before revascularization[12] by coronary artery bypass graft became the standard of care revealed a poor prognosis for these patients, with a three-year survival rate as low as 37 percent.

Acute total occlusion of LMCA is a highly morbid clinical event, and it is one of the leading causes of sudden cardiac death (SCD)—"a widow maker."

After the test, I looked at Pete and reflected for a moment on his nonfaith. There had to be some invisible force that was protecting him. Time was wasted between debating the merits of atheism and the HMO's stonewalling. It was a miracle that he was still alive. The size of the LMCA was reduced from a cigarette butt to a thin strand. The bulk of the blood supply to his heart was coming through this miniscule lifeline. He came very close to dying from a heart attack; I did not know how Pete would feel about God after this watershed event. From my demeanor and eye contact, he realized that he was in deep trouble.

"Big problem?" he asked.

"Yes, you will need urgent bypass surgery," I said softly. He closed his eyes for a moment and accepted my recommendation.

I spoke to the cardiac surgeon, and Pete was put on the Operating Room schedule.

The next day before the operation when I entered his room, I was pleasantly surprised to see him sitting in the chair in a Buddhist meditation posture; both eyes were closed, the right hand rested atop the left, and the thumbs were touching. It is said that one's meditation will not be good if one's posture is not good. He was surrounded by three Buddhist monks who were chanting the mantra to the white umbrella goddess—Buddha of Protection.

Looking at Pete (an atheist) in this contemplative and spiritual posture, I was observing a fundamental total transformation, a metamorphosis—the emergence of a new man from the ashes of the old. After the end of prayer when Pete opened his eyes, he was surprised to find me sitting in the room and waiting to teach him the postop breathing exercises. He apologized, but I assured him that he needed all the help—both spiritual and nonspiritual—to get through this surgery. I thanked the monks for their mantras and blessings. Pete was wheeled into surgery.

When I came out of his room, the head nurse dashed across the corridor and told me that Pete's wife, Nancy, was waiting for me in the conference room.

"Were you surprised to see Pete praying with the monks?" she asked when I entered the room.

"I was, because when I met Pete for the first time in the office, he told me that he is an atheist," I replied.

"You must have heard the popular aphorism, '*There are no atheists in foxholes*,' and Pete may turn out to be one of them," she said.

"Nancy, *there are many atheists in foxholes*." I defended Pete because it would have been rude to question his faith. A well-known study published in the *European Journal of Personality* shows that strong atheists and strong religious believers reveal a low level of death anxiety, whereas in a time of crisis, nonreligious participants are more inclined toward religious belief. The nonreligious participants and weak atheists suffer more from death anxiety. So, a weak atheist may not stay an atheist at the time of personal crisis. I was not sure about Pete, whether he was a weak or a strong atheist. Only time would tell.

Nancy continued, "My interest in Buddhism has been lifelong, dating from my teens when I read Hermann Hesse's novel *Siddhartha*, but only in the last ten years have I really had the opportunity to seriously pursue this interest.

"I was raised in the Protestant church and certainly benefited from the values and morals that those teachings instilled in me. Yet, by the time I was in my midteens during the turbulent era that began in the 1960s, I was deeply disturbed by my church's reluctance to address any of the significant social and political issues that were facing the country. My commitment to social activism overrode any loyalty to the church, from which I resigned, never to return."

"When did you become a Buddhist?" I asked.

She continued, "When the Buddhist vihara was established on the property next door to us, I quickly saw it as an opportunity to direct my vague interest in Buddhism into more intense study and involvement. I have been involved in weekly group meditation and *Dhamma* talk sessions, attended *pujas*, provided *dana* periodically to the monks, and attended many religious functions at the vihara."

"What about Pete? Did he participate in the *Dhamma* sessions?" I asked.

"Pete, my husband, was always an atheist at heart, and did not share my interest in Buddhism. He and I were both committed to helping the monks get established and assisting in the many projects that were going on. The monks were always there to lend a hand in helping us out as well," she said.

"While building the Buddha statue, the monks had failed to get a structural steel inspection before pouring the substructure concrete. The township inspector was to come out and close down the construction. The monks asked Pete to speak to him. He testified and assured them that the substructure was sound. To the amusement of the monks and the inspector, Pete told the inspector that the only thing that could bring down the structure was either an earthquake that measured eight on the Richter scale or the Taliban, which to the best of his knowledge were not operating in New Jersey. The inspector was surprisingly amused and decided not to issue a stop-work order. As the monks were always there to lend a hand in helping us out, they chose Pete as the first symbolic greeter when Maha-thera [a monk who has been in the order for more than twenty years] made his official visit to the temple."

Pete's surgery was uneventful and without complication. The monks from the vihara came to visit every day that he was convalescing in the hospital to pray for his recovery. After a short stay in rehab, he went home to recuperate.

One month after surgery, Pete came back to the office for follow-up.

"Pete, the EKG is back to normal, and looking at it, nobody could tell that you had major heart surgery," I complimented him.

"Thanks," he replied.

"Pete, do you believe that the positive outcome of surgery was influenced by the monks' intervention?" I looked at him intently. "You came very close to suffering a fatal heart attack. Some divine power must have protected you."

He looked at me but kept quiet, reflecting on and analyzing my question.

I continued, "Nancy told me about you and the Buddhist vihara. You, an atheist, helping the monks to establish a Buddhist temple!"

"I am an atheist, not an orthodox Christian or Reverend Rick Warren," he replied.

"What do you mean?" I asked.

"Reverend Rick Warren's book, *The Purpose-Driven Life*, is a huge success because he recognizes our need for a purpose beyond centeredness. He writes that he has seen many nominally religious or nonreligious people who are struggling with a sense of purposelessness today, even as they gain in both scientific knowledge and material prosperity. 'The man without a purpose is like a ship without a rudder—a waif, a nothing, a no man.' Warren argues forcefully that 'It's not about you,' insisting that life and society are at best when we overcome selfishness and learn to live for a purpose higher than ourselves."

He continued, "Unfortunately, Warren's idea about a purposeful life is nothing more than packaging orthodox Christianity in a humanistic box. He writes with entirely God-given confidence that life's higher purpose can only be Christianity as interpreted by people like him, and that those who disagree will spend eternity in hell, 'apart from God forever.' It is sad to see people like him so openly prejudiced against those who agree with him about the need for purpose but prefer Islam, Judaism, or any other simple humanist faith."("Good without God" by Greg Epstein).

He concluded, "There is no way to prove that the positive outcome of heart surgery was influenced by the monks' interventions, but I feel certain it was significant. I was born and raised in the Christian faith. I became an atheist, but after the bypass surgery I will end my journey as an agnostic. I hope my circle is complete—faith—no faith—faith."

He looked at me. I noticed a unique kindness and peace in his eyes, indicating that finally he discovered his God by reaffirming his faith in altruism and humanism through helping the monks make a home for themselves in the God-blessed United States.

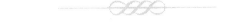

THE CARDIAC TRANSPLANT

I met Mike in summer 1998 when he came to the office for a
cardiac evaluation. "The new patient is very sick. Please see
him first," the nurse alerted me.

Mike was a forty-two-year-old male with a friendly, round
face and dusky complexion; he was sweating profusely, sitting
on the edge of the table, and struggling to breathe. He was not
able to lie flat due to nocturnal dyspnea[13] and had been sleeping
on the recliner. He had suffered a massive heart attack about
two months ago and was admitted to the hospital. The doctor
told him that he was not a suitable candidate for heart surgery.

On his patient demographic and medical history form, Mike
said that he had been having difficulty breathing, which was
progressively getting worse. The symptoms started about two
weeks prior. First, he had experienced angina-like chest pain on
walking, and then he'd had episodes of near-syncope (fainting)
while climbing a flight of stairs.

Mike introduced his wife, who was standing next to him.

"How long has he been having this breathing problem?" I asked.

"Since the heart attack. He won't go back to see the hospital cardiologist. Our neighbor, who is your patient, recommended you," his wife said.

"What kind of tests did he have after the heart attack?" I asked.

His wife, Mary, gave me a brief history. "He had been in good health except minor aches and pains. He was awakened from sleep with chest pressure and heartburn that would not go away with Maalox®. We finally decided to go to the hospital. The doctors in the hospital told us that he'd had a major heart attack. Next day, the doctor did a heart catheterization, which showed that all the major coronary arteries were blocked. The doctor said he'd waited too long at home without getting the proper treatment. The heart muscle was damaged, and there was nothing he could do to repair the heart."

"What kind of doctor tells the patient that 'nothing can be done'?" Mike asked. "I have no confidence in the doctor, and that's why I will not go back to see him."

I agreed with him. No doctor should ever tell the patient that "there is nothing that can be done." It is hard to tell a sick patient that there is no hope of getting better.

Clearly, there was no meaningful communication between Mike and the hospital cardiologist. The patient-doctor relationship is built on certain expectations from both parties. If the patient has fair expectations from the doctor to be informed and educated about the illness, and if the doctor has not met those expectations, then an effective relationship between doctor and patient will never develop.

Patient-doctor communication is the most crucial factor that will lead either to a therapeutic or a harmful relationship. This communication is both verbal as well as nonverbal, and if the patient feels that the doctor has violated his or her dignity or was disrespectful, then he or she will not develop enough trust in the doctor.

Most patients are nervous meeting the doctor for the first time. So, while taking patient history, the doctor should give ample opportunity for patients to talk about themselves. This helps the physician to know and understand patients and their inner core, psyche, pains, and fears; it is the person the doctor is treating, not the disease.

The dynamics of communication between patients and their doctors have changed dramatically with the introduction of technology. According to Dr. Harlan Krumholz, "The loss of respect for the power of connecting with the patient is not the fault of doctors, but seems to be a by-product of the medical environment that we have created. Doctors lose when relationships are a casualty of the production mentality that focuses intently on relative value unit (RVU),[15] the currency of medical output, rather than the results achieved with patients—including the nature of the relationship."(Wall Street Journal 12 April, 2013)

The infinite worth of a caring doctor is being corrupted and degraded into RVUs. The total RVU has three components: work (RVUw), practice expense (RVUpE), and malpractice (RVUmp). These units determine the reimbursement for the medical procedures doctors perform. There are no RVUs for empathy, compassion, and communication for doctors, so why bother? The future of medicine is on a slippery slope, and judging the worth of a doctor with RVUs is destroying the soul of our profession.

This system of reimbursement has pitted specialty against specialty. The art of medicine and doctors' thinking have become hostage to RVUs (currency of medical output). I think "Independence Day" will come—the day Medicare abolishes this monstrosity that is degrading the medical profession.

The relationship between a doctor and the patient is built on mutual trust and proper communication. In medical school, most of our time is spent on learning the pathophysiology, treatment, and prognosis of life-threatening diseases, but there is no time for learning the art of communication. The skill to connect with patients and understand their pain requires a unique kind of intelligence.

In 1995, Daniel Goleman's best-selling book, *Emotional Intelligence: Why It Can Matter More Than IQ*, further elaborates the role of emotions in personal and professional growth. After publication of this book, the term *EI* became very popular and created much discord among psychologists.

According to Goleman's model, there are main EI constructs such as self-awareness, self-regulation, social skills, empathy, and motivation (being driven to achieve for the sake of achievement).

Is EI innate, or is it learned capabilities? Can we teach a person to be emotionally competent? I don't think so. We can't teach a person to be empathetic and kind to other people's suffering. EI is a blessing from God. Either you have it or you don't.

Most doctors are smart; studying and understanding complex heart conditions require doctors to be intelligent and knowledgeable. Facing death and sickness, however, requires more than book knowledge. It demands special skills—God's gift of EI.

A doctor who applies the right combination of IQ and EQ (emotional quotient) while taking care of patients will help patients not only get well but also heal normally after a life-threatening illness.

"The doctor in the hospital who told us there was nothing he could do devastated my husband. Our family was whipsawed by that emotional event," Mary said.

"We have three kids: one son and two daughters. I've been working overtime to build a nest for the family. Although the heart attack shattered my dreams, I was hopeful that the doctor would help me to heal and get back on my feet," Mike added.

"What kind of work do you do?" I asked.

"I'm a roofer and work for a small-sized company," Mike said.

I saw the pain and anguish on his face. What hurt him the most—the heart attack or the doctor's thoughtless comments?

In Mike, a sick patient, I saw a deficit of hope and an abundance of pain and suffering. He was desperately seeking *hope* more than the pills. My job was to balance the treatment and give him hope and the will to live. This was the front-burner issue for me, not the pills or high-tech cardiac procedures. The effect of pills is subtherapeutic without the proper mind-set.

The thinking process and physical healing are as intimately connected as fire and heat—we cannot separate them.

Hope is the doorway that brings in the rays of light and aids in expecting wholeness around the corner. The patient's life resembles a dark tunnel riddled with pain, suffering, and fear. The physicians whom the sick employ in their helplessness should be mindful of this fact; they have a moral and ethical responsibility not to shut this doorway to hope.

I had to educate Mike about his sickness before dealing with the physical aspect of his illness.

I said, "Biology is inherently variable."

It is extremely difficult for a cardiologist to predict the long-term prognosis of a patient after a heart attack. Every person is born with his or her own *internal healing clock*. After a major illness like a heart attack, the patient has to change his or her lifestyle to protect this clock.

We can diagnose heart attacks, but no test is available to evaluate what kind of *healing processes* a patient has inherited. After a massive heart attack, some patients recover promptly and lead a normal life because by changing their lifestyle they have tuned up the healing processes. Other patients continue to smoke and eat unhealthy food, which will slow down the healing clock and will prolong their recovery from a major heart attack.

What makes a difference between life and death is not only the nature of the disease, but also the conditioning of our unique internal healing clock.

I continued, "The time to fight a major illness is when you're healthy—that is, leading a healthy lifestyle—not when you're sick. A healthy lifestyle, which includes diet, exercise, as well as reflection and meditation with a touch of spirituality, will keep the healing clock humming. That is why I never tell patients 'nothing can be done.'"

It is safe for doctors to be pessimistic about the prognosis because the burden of failed optimism and its emotional consequences for family members would be too heavy to carry. According to Dr. Jerome Groopman in *The Anatomy of Hope*, "When the physician feels that he or she really cannot do anything active, they tend to take the most negative scenario as the likely one. It is easier to give people the worst news and then if something good comes about, everyone is overjoyed."

Mike looked at me and smiled. I saw a ray of hope on his face that vanished abruptly when his wife said, "He continues to smoke."

"I promise not to smoke ever again," he said. I was surprised when he took the pack of cigarettes from his pocket and threw it in the garbage can.

On physical examination, the sweating of his face and his breathing difficulty had lessened. After our conversation, I think he became less nervous and more relaxed.

His heart rate was 88 beats per minute, blood pressure was 115/60, and his respiratory rate was seventeen breaths per minute. He had distended neck veins and basilar rales in both lungs.

On cardiac examination, his heart rhythm was regular with normal S1 and S2 that split during expiration. There was an S4 gallop at the apex with a pansystolic murmur radiating to the axilla. No diastolic murmur was appreciated. The carotid upstroke was diminished.

The EKG showed a regular sinus rhythm with a large, old anterolateral myocardial infarction.[16] A limited echocardiogram showed that the internal dimensions of the left ventricle had markedly increased with a large apical aneurysm. Color Doppler showed mitral valve[17] and tricuspid valve insufficiency.[18] There was a significant decrease in the left ventricle systolic function.

Mike was suffering from class II–III congestive heart failure,[19] which is produced when the heart is unable to meet the metabolic needs of the body while maintaining normal ventricular filling pressures. His symptoms of congestive heart failure were due to a combination of forward failure[20] (low cardiac output) as well as backward failure (increased filling pressures). The cause of congestive heart failure in his case was the heart attack, which interrupted the blood supply and damaged the heart muscle.

Heart failure is a chronic progressive disease and carries a bad prognosis. The annual mortality rate varies from 20 percent to 60 percent, and death associated with congestive heart failure may occur suddenly (sudden cardiac death) or from cardiogenic shock[21] and end-organ failure.

After the cardiac examination, I asked Mike and Mary to come to the consultation room to further discuss the treatment plan. This kind of meeting would give me insight and the opportunity to evaluate the dynamics of their relationship as husband and wife. I believe that after a major illness, a marriage has a tremendous therapeutic or toxic effect on the outcome and prognosis.

"What's wrong? Why is he having difficulty in breathing?" Mary asked.

"Mike is suffering from chronic congestive heart failure, which is making it difficult for him to breathe. The pumping chambers of the heart are damaged, and the heart is not able to pump all the blood it gets. This leads to high pressure in the lungs and causes labored breathing and fatigue." I explained to Mary the complex pathophysiology of heart failure in the simplest words she could relate to so that she could understand the disease.

"Am I going to continue to suffer like this?" Mike asked. "The doctor said there was nothing he could do."

"The hospital doctor told you that—not me," I pointed out. "I have three major treatment goals to achieve to relieve the breathing difficulty and prevent more damage to the heart, but the most important goal is getting you back on your feet so you can take care of your family. I will not succeed in this mission without your cooperation," I said.

"It'd be insane not to follow your instructions. You just saw me throw away my cigarettes," he said.

"Relapse in congestive heart failure frequently occurs and has serious consequences. Poor treatment compliance is very common in patients with congestive heart failure. There will have to be major lifestyle changes, like eating a low-salt diet, abstaining from alcohol, quitting smoking, and reducing psychological stress. These are precipitating factors that trigger the relapse of congestive heart failure," I explained.

His new medicine list included an angiotensin-receptor blocker (ARB), a beta-blocker (carvedilol), and a diuretic (bumetanide). I added two more pills, spironolactone and digoxin, to his treatment regimen.

"The salt restriction is the most important and mandatory; it reduces the volume overload and relieves the symptoms of congestive heart failure. A low-sodium diet includes no more than two to three thousand milligrams of sodium. To give you an idea of how much that is, one teaspoonful of salt is approximately twenty-three hundred milligrams of sodium. Mike, you should limit your sodium intake to about two thousand milligrams, or one teaspoon, per day," I explained.

The low-salt diet is as important as pills in patients with congestive heart failure; I have seen stable and well-controlled congestive heart failure patients go into pulmonary edema[22] (acute heart failure) after eating a corned beef sandwich and potato chips. It is a dangerous pairing for patients with congestive heart failure.

Mike looked at me and said, "Dr. Kumar, I'm Italian. This low-salt diet is for a rabbit, not for an Italian man who grew up with ham, prosciutto, and salami."

Mary looked at him sharply. She did not appreciate the humor in his statement. "He reaches for the salt shaker without tasting the food, and it worries me that he will not follow the diet."

I replied, "A total of seventy-seven percent of salt eaten comes from processed foods and restaurant foods, and eleven percent from the dining table. The rest is found naturally in foodstuffs. Not buying processed foods and eliminating table salt will reduce our salt intake by eighty-eight percent." Then I added, "It's up to Mike to decide and pick either a low-salt diet or congestive heart failure." I reinforced the issue because without lifestyle modifications, he would never come out of congestive heart failure and would die prematurely.

I was aware of my own limitations, worried that I might have given him false hope, because I did not know the result of the tests he'd had in the hospital. Without the evaluation of cardiac data, his clinical assessment was incomplete. However, I was successful in establishing rapport and the beginning of a mutually trusting relationship.

The most important part of treatment is the education of patients about a high-salt diet and its harmful effect on congestive heart failure. The high-tech invasive procedures that I would recommend to him would be less effective if there were no lifestyle modifications and dietary sodium restrictions.

Mike's journey to healing after such a devastating illness would be long and painful. On his way to recovery, I knew he would encounter many painful bumps of disappointments and false expectations.

The initial management of congestive heart failure, spending a lot of time in explaining high-tech intervention and not educating the patient about lifestyle modifications, is like putting the cart before the horse. The evaluation of cardiac data was important, but at this first visit, I wanted to help him to start his journey on the right track.

"Mary, I would like Mike to sign the form giving me permission to get his medical records from the hospital for further evaluation. The salt-restricted diet will not change, whatever the hospital records show," I said. (I reemphasized the importance of diet.)

The hospital records showed that he was admitted with pulmonary edema (acute left heart failure) due to massive anterior wall myocardial infarction. He was intubated and treated with massive dosages of diuretics. The echocardiogram done in the Cardiac Care Unit (CCU) showed ejection fraction of 35 percent (55–70 percent). Miraculously, his recovery was as dramatic as his sickness. He was extubated within forty-eight hours and transferred out of CCU.

The cardiac catheterization was done to evaluate the extent of coronary artery disease and the severity of mitral valve regurgitation. The catheterization showed that he was suffering from diffuse blockage in the distal coronary arteries with moderate mitral regurgitation. There were no focal areas of stenosis where the surgeon could hook the coronary artery bypass grafts (CABG)[23].

In patients who are suffering from coronary artery disease, "the anatomy decides the destiny" and, obviously, Mike's coronary arteries were diffusely diseased and were not suitable for CABG. He was a sick man with young kids and limited treatment options.

⚬⚬⚬

"Mary is taking her husband to the emergency room because he is having dizzy spells and difficulty breathing," my nurse informed me.

Mike did not respond to oral diuretics and went in pulmonary edema (acute heart failure). The ER physician at Robert Wood Johnson (RWJ) University Hospital started him on intravenous (IV) diuretics and called me to discuss further management and a treatment plan. I was relieved to know that Mike was in RWJ because he would need advanced, sophisticated cardiac testing, which was available there.

The history of RWJ University Hospital is remarkable. In a short time, it has evolved from a small community hospital to a top-ranked institution in delivering cardiothoracic care. This institution has not abandoned its social purpose of caring for the sick and disadvantaged.

It was established in 1885 as New Brunswick City Hospital. In 1888, the medical directors raised $3,000 to purchase land for the John Wells Memorial Hospital. In 1916, the name was changed to Middlesex General Hospital. In January 1986, the president of the university announced that effective that coming July 1, the UMDNJ–Rutgers Medical School in Piscataway and Middlesex General Hospital in New Brunswick would be renamed UMDNJ–RWJ Medical School and RWJ University Hospital.

Mike was admitted to the CCU and started on IV medications to strengthen his heart. The blood tests showed that he suffered a minor heart attack that damaged more heart muscle. The review of the nuclear cardiac scan showed a large anteroapical aneurysm with moderately severe mitral regurgitation.

Mike was responding to medications, and the cardiac failure was stable. However, it was obvious that the medications were not the answer to his life-threatening disease. This cardiac stability was an illusion. If we waited too long, the next heart attack could turn out to be fatal. I had no options except to work expeditiously, not wasting precious time by trying different medications.

Next morning, I presented his case at a cardiothoracic conference. The cardiac data were analyzed by cardiac surgeons and a group of cardiologists; different treatment options were debated and rejected.

Patients are not aware that doctors spend countless hours behind the scenes to make the right treatment decisions. We cardiologists work on the presumption of *zero error* because a little neglect or a misstep can have devastating consequences. The cardiothoracic conference is specifically designed to discuss all the treatment options, and once consensus is reached, cardiac surgery is recommended to the patient. Our mission at RWJ University Hospital is to meet the zero-error goal in cardiothoracic surgery.

The final treatment recommendation for Mike was a cardiac transplant as he was not a candidate for coronary bypass surgery. A cardiac transplant was the only treatment option to save his life. Medications would relieve his symptoms but would not prolong his life. Without a cardiac transplant, the prognosis was grave. A one-year mortality rate was more than 50 percent.

After the conference, I went to see Mike and found him sitting on the chair reading the newspaper. He had no complaints of chest pain or difficulty in breathing. The inotropes[24] and diuretics[25] did a wonderful job. On examination, the lungs were dry, not congested, and the blood oxygen saturation was normal.

"How do you feel?" I asked.

"I feel good—no more chest pressure or breathing difficulty. The medications you gave did this miracle," he said.

"Thanks," I said.

"I hope that soon I will be able to go back to work," he said.

"Mike, when your wife comes, let the nurse know so we can discuss further treatment options," I said, and left the room to continue morning rounds.

The irony of the situation was that he was worrying about going back to work, and I was agonizing over how to tell him without wasting precious time that the only viable option was a cardiac transplant. I had to give him the bad news that he was not fit to go back to work and that he needed a new heart to survive. I had to be careful with my words so that he did not get disheartened and depressed but rather, would stay optimistic about the future and not give up. I knew that if he lost hope, I would lose him. Depression and anxiety are two of the many causes of cardiac arrhythmia[26] and death in patients like Mike who are suffering from end-stage ischemic cardiomyopathy.[27]

Mike's cardiac condition was stable, and I told the nurse to call me when his wife came to see him. I wanted his wife to be in the room when I told him about the heart surgery. It is well known that when a husband and wife tackle an illness together, it is easier to keep a positive outlook. Couples who know that they are going through this as a team may be less stressed and worried. I was hoping that the presence of his wife would give him an emotional anchor to hold on to.

"This morning I had a conference with a group of cardiac surgeons and other cardiologists, and we looked at all the tests Mike has gone through. The medications that are helping now will stop working eventually. This medical treatment is not the final answer. Mike will need more than medications to get well and go back to work," I said.

"What is the final verdict? Before, the doctors told me nothing can be done," Mike said.

"You will need a cardiac transplant because the damage to the heart muscle is extensive, and no minor repair or bypass will help you to get well," I said.

I looked at his face for his reaction to the information and was pleasantly surprised to see that there was a glimmer of hope in his eyes and a quiet resolve on his face, indicating that he was ready to fight and get well. His wife stood up with teary eyes and reached for his hand. She held it against her face. She quietly sobbed, letting the bright, shining tears fall on his hand. No words were exchanged between husband and wife. Time stood still. This act of compassion and kindness needed no verbal validation; the emotional impact of this act was too powerful to describe.

It is the compassion between husband and wife that nurtures the roots of their marriage. At a time of crisis, these strong roots that have been cultivated by love and kindness will not let the marriage fall apart. I was happy to see that Mike's marriage would stand the test of time, and his wife's kindness and compassion would help him to beat the odds and get well.

War is the only proper school for surgeons.
—HIPPOCRATES

The Hippocratic Oath is based on the principle of beneficence: "for the benefit of the sick according to [the physician's] ability and judgment."

For much of recorded history, doctors saw the human heart as a throbbing seat of the soul, a unique gift from God, too delicate to tinker with.

During World War II, military doctors were able to experiment with anesthesia and other elements of modern surgery.

Surgeons were able to remove bullets and pieces of shrapnel from the chest but were unable to do major repairs on the heart. The major stumbling block to doing heart surgery was the time factor, because the interruption of circulation for more than four minutes would cause irreversible brain damage.

That changed in 1953 when Dr. John H. Gibbon Jr. of Philadelphia used a heart-lung respirator to keep an eighteen-year-old patient alive for twenty-seven minutes while he repaired the hole in her heart. This invention paved the way for open heart surgery to enter widespread use.

<hr />

The first successful heart transplants were from one frog to another frog and then one dog to another dog. The leap to a human recipient took place in the 1960s when a team of surgeons in Jackson, Mississippi, performed the first chimpanzee-to-human cardiac transplant. Mr. Boyd Rush was the first human recipient of a chimpanzee's heart. Boyd died ninety minutes after his transplant. This failure revealed that surgeons had to use human hearts if transplants were to achieve long-term success.

The dream and possibility of human-to-human heart transplants lived on.

In 1967, Dr. Christiaan Barnard of South Africa performed the first human-to-human cardiac transplant, sewing the heart of a young woman killed in a car accident into the chest of a middle-aged man. After four hours of surgery, a single jolt of electricity started it beating. "Christ," Barnard said, "it is going to work."

The patient survived the surgery, but the immunosuppressants weakened him. Eighteen days after the operation, he succumbed to pneumonia and died.

Each year, heart failure affects 7.5 million patients in the United States. Recent data show that 5 percent to 10 percent of all patients with heart failure have advanced disease that is associated with high mortality. In the most advanced phase of heart failure, a heart transplant has been the only means of improving the quality of life and survival in these patients. A heart transplant is available to only a fraction of those who need it because of the shortage of available donors.

The patients have to go through elaborate preselection testing in order to make the transplant list. Mike would be put on the priority list for a transplant because of his relatively young age and no history of chronic diseases.

———— ∞ ————

"Where will I go for the heart transplant?" Mike asked.

"We will do the transplant at RWJ University Hospital." I deliberately used the word *we* and not *you* to give him the message that he was not alone in this battle; there would be many good and caring people working behind the scenes to get him through this ordeal.

Deemed suitable for the transplant, Mike was discharged from the hospital on oral medications. His response to intravenous inotropes was dramatic because of good cardiac reserve, but this improvement in heart failure would not last. It was a temporary phenomenon, an eerie calm before the storm.

"I'm glad to go home because I have a few legal things to take care of," Mike said.

Mike's congestive heart failure was stable on his follow-up examinations; this was a welcome development that did not surprise me. I had seen this kind of response with other patients who'd had a brief but dramatic response after a short course of intravenous inotropes. These medications tune up the tired and partially dead heart muscles, unmasking the cardiac reserve, which can improve the function of the heart. This was temporary relief. Mike was happy and eager to get back to work, but I advised him to go on disability. He was not fit to fix people's broken roofs when his own heart was broken. My treatment objective was to stretch this salutary effect of cardiac reserve as much as possible and delay the transplant. The close monitoring of medications and a proper low-salt diet were helping him to stay out of congestive heart failure.

More than six months later, Mike's congestive heart failure was still stable. He was regular in his follow-up visits with me and the congestive heart failure clinic. Although things were stable, I knew that this was an organized instability. A little carelessness with diet or medications would put him back into heart failure.

"I may go to prison," Mike said when I saw him in the office during a routine follow-up.

"What?" I wasn't sure whether I'd heard him correctly.

"I have been out of work for the last nine months, and to make extra money, I did a few dumb things and got caught. In three weeks, I will be facing the judge for a final hearing," he said.

"Why didn't you tell me you were going through all this?" I asked.

"I was embarrassed and worried that after knowing about the criminal acts I've done, you'd decide not to care for me," he said.

Although Mike had left the office, his words *going to jail* were still ringing in my head. Without proper medical care, he would not survive even a brief period of incarceration. I had been taking care of him for the last several months, and during his admission to the hospital, I'd met his family, his mother, and his brother—hardworking, decent people. He was not a hard-core criminal but a victim of circumstances and bad luck. Most likely, his motivation was to protect his family from the ravages of financial hardship. Doctors are advised to stay out of a patient's private life, and the prevailing teaching in modern medicine is a patient's autonomy. However, sometimes, a paternalistic act to help the patient becomes the "moral obligation" of the doctor. To protect the patient is a "sacred duty" of the doctor—it is the foundation of our covenant with God.

Mike did not ask for help, but my feeling of paternalism prevailed. My desire to protect him compelled me to write on his behalf the following letter to the judge without his knowledge:

Dear Judge _____,

I am writing this letter on behalf of Mr. _____, whose case will soon come before you for sentencing. I am a cardiologist, currently licensed in the State of New Jersey.

It has come to my attention that Mr. _____ has been charged with certain crimes that, if he is found guilty, would result in incarceration for an extended period of time. Mr. _____ currently suffers from end-stage ischemic cardiomyopathy and class IV congestive heart failure and has been under my care for the last nine months. As a result of his condition, he requires regular monitoring of the medications. These medications have life-threatening side effects and need to be adjusted frequently.

Mr. _____'s condition is severe and requires a significant level of medical care and expertise; I have put him on highly complicated, tailor-made, specific medical care. He is on a strict low-salt diet with close monitoring for weight gain; his medications are adjusted according to his weight on a weekly basis. I think that incarcerating him would deprive him of access to proper medical care. I cannot comment or make any determination regarding Mr. _____'s culpability with respect to the crime that he is charged with. I do not purport to have any expertise in the law. I strongly believe that those who break or otherwise violate the law should be punished accordingly, and in proportion to the crime committed. However, in my opinion, any verdict resulting in Mr. _____'s incarceration would deprive him of proper medical care and would be tantamount to the death penalty.

As a physician, it is my duty to act in the best interest of my patient. This duty is immortalized in the Hippocratic Oath we take when we are awarded our medical degree, and it governs the conduct of our profession. I would like to reiterate that I write to you without Mr. _____'s knowledge and humbly request that you consider Mr. _____'s condition when delivering your judgment.

Best regards,

Ashok Kumar, MD

Thank God, Mike was not incarcerated but put under house arrest with an ankle bracelet for two months. He was allowed to continue his medical treatment. Soon after the end of the parole period, he was readmitted to RWJ University Hospital with worsening congestive heart failure. He was a lucky man because while still in the hospital and on inotropes, a matching heart became available. It was the heart of a young man who died in a motorbike accident. After the cardiac transplant, Mike was transferred to a rehab center and discharged after two weeks of physiotherapy.

MOLECULES OF EMOTION

"Can the heart transplant change my husband's personality?" Nancy asked when she and Mike came to see me for a follow-up. "Before the operation he hated desserts and would not go near the computer, but now he craves sweets and spends most of his time on the Internet." She was concerned about her husband's changed behavior and wanted to know that there was no complication affecting the brain during surgery.

"I think the heart transplant is more than replacing an organ that no longer functions. The heart is the source of love and emotions and the center that houses feelings and forms the personality," I said. I had no scientifically valid explanation to answer her question. I assured her that Mike's surgery was without complications.

"A family friend knew the donor, and upon meeting the 'family of his heart,' we discovered that the donor was a computer programmer," she said.

"I think the donor's soul is living in my new heart," Mike insisted, "because when the heart was removed from the donor, all the nerves were separated and cut. It takes time for nerves to regenerate, but how come soon after surgery I started having all kinds of feelings for my wife and a craving for sweets? As my wife said, I hated sweets before the heart transplant. The donor's heart remembers all the good things he loved. He is gone, but I think his heart and his soul are living in me." I looked at Mike and found him sitting in a pensive and reflective mood, contemplating the mysteries of his new heart. "I hope the immunotherapy will not destroy this gentle soul that I have inherited from the donor," he whispered.

Mike's observation was correct, and he was trying to explain to me a unique phenomenon we see in heart transplants called cellular memory phenomenon.

In a study published in the *Journal of Quality of Life Research*, researchers found that 6 percent of heart transplant patients noticed a drastic change in their personality due to their new heart. These patients seem to be more susceptible to something called cellular memory phenomenon. The cellular memory is not 100 percent scientifically validated, but its presence in patients after a heart transplant is difficult to brush aside.

Cellular memory is defined as the idea that the cells in our body contain the information about taste and personality. Every cell in our body has its own mind, and if we transfer tissues from one body to another, the cells from the first body will carry memories to the second body.

Some scientists believe that cellular memory does exist. Dr. Candace Pert, a biochemist, found that the brain and the body send messages to each other through short-chain amino acids known as neuropeptides. These amino acid chains were previously known to exist exclusively in the brain; however, Dr. Pert has found them in major organs like the heart. The role of these neuropeptides in cellular memory is being debated but has not been proved.

Another scientist, Dr. J. Andrew Armour, attempts to explain the concept of cellular memory through a new discipline in cardiology called neuroradiology. According to Dr. Armour, the communication between the brain and the heart is a two-way dialogue. The heart has its own intrinsic nervous system that he calls a "little brain in the heart." In his book *Neurocardiology*, Dr. Armour states that the intrinsic nervous system functions independently of the brain and nervous system at large. This allows the transplanted heart to work like a normal heart both physically and emotionally, even when all the nerves are severed.

Ancient cultures, too, have talked about the metaphysical heart—the heart that shows us the difference between simply living and actually feeling alive. *Huang Di Nei Jing* is the oldest medical book to originate from China. It was written by numerous authors. From this ancient classic came the foundations of traditional Chinese medicine (TCM). TCM is believed to have been practiced as early as 471–221 BCE.

In TCM, the Zang-Fu Theory explains the concept of cellular memory in the human body. The organs that can be transplanted—the heart, lung, liver, spleen, and kidney—are called zang organs. Not only do these organs have strong cellular memory, but they also have feelings and emotions.

Heart Joy Shen (Mind)
Lung Grief Po (Corporeal Soul)
Liver Anger Hun (Ethereal Soul)
Spleen Pensiveness Yi (Intellect)
Kidney Fear Zhi (Will)

The fu organs do not have a strong cellular memory.

According to ancient Hindu texts, memory is everywhere, in each particle of our body, and it is recorded in the prana (life force).

Food is imbued with the consciousness of the cook; a mother's cooking is always delicious. Hindus believe that along with a piece of meat, you swallow a little consciousness of the dead animal you eat. These metaphysical concepts about cellular memory in the meat of dead animals might have compelled ancient India to go vegetarian and give to the world the "science of meditation."

When heart transplant patients describe the enigma of cellular memory with metaphysical explanations, we should not brush aside their concerns. The essential point is that the cells in our body are ruled by forces and powers far larger than we understand. Therefore, we should keep an open mind.

After Mike's cardiac transplant, I did not allow him to go back to his old job of fixing people's roofs. His newly acquired passion for computers through cellular memory became his asset. He went back to college and graduated as a computer programmer. He lived almost twenty years after his cardiac transplant and died from hepatic failure.

The following letter describes a similar incident experienced by another of my cardiac transplant patients after his operation:

Hello, Dr. Kumar:

This is a follow-up to my discussion with you regarding my postop observation.

Let me briefly walk you through my thoughts, feelings, and perceptions.

My cardiac transplant was done on January 19, 2014, at Newark Beth Israel Medical Center. I must say my experience there has been positive. The staff knew what they were doing. After the operation, the doctor told my son that the heart donor was from New Jersey and was twenty-nine years old. That is the only information she could give us. I am going to describe my feelings aside from the side effects of medicines.

Dr. Kumar, you have been my doctor for more than twenty-five years. I consider you to be a very unique doctor whose approach is quite significant compared to that of other doctors I know. You are a thinker outside the norm and have a vast knowledge of metaphysics. You are open to any and all possibilities. You treat the patient, not the disease. That is why I am describing how I have been feeling without the risk of making it a laughing matter.

Ever since I got home after a two-week hospital stay, I have been feeling different.

My behavior as the time progressed changed in subtle ways. My taste toward food changed dramatically. Preoperatively, I had been a meat-and-potatoes guy who had to have meat every day. I did not like vegetables like Brussels sprouts, broccoli, cauliflower, etc. But now I do not yearn for meat or rice. I prefer vegetables and beans/legumes. My food portions are small and reduced to 25 percent of [their] pre-op portions. The same is true with bread and main courses. Pre-op I would eat one big serving for the entire day, but now I can only eat little portions several times a day. I cannot watch action or horror shows/movies anymore. Instead, romantic comedies appeal to me more. When I am about to open a beverage bottle cap, my thought is to get help because I won't be able to open it. I am a lot less aggressive while driving, or if I am having a conversation or texting, I do not raise my voice to assert my point anymore. My entire outlook toward the world and the environment have changed in subtle ways as if I have more feminine emotions, which were not present pre-op.

Because of these unusual feelings, I mentioned to my son that I think my new heart is affecting my behavior, and we need to confirm if I have a woman's heart. He laughed about it but agreed to somehow find out the gender of my heart donor. During my next follow-up visit, we found out that indeed it is a woman's heart. I leave it to you to determine if indeed my feelings and observations are realistic or not. Personally I am convinced that the heart of another human does bring characteristics of the original owner. It is up to the sensitivity of the new owner whether he or she can feel the subtle changes.

I look forward to having you as my doctor for another twenty-five years; frankly, I would not have survived this long without your ever-so-careful treatment. In my eyes you are not just a doctor but a healer as well.

Thank you for everything, including a very timely recommendation of my heart transplant.

Most scientists and doctors believe that cellular memory exists metaphysically, but they are extremely uncomfortable talking about it. There is no valid scientific explanation to describe this phenomenon.

For those patients who are experiencing this mystic phenomenon, my advice is not to get alarmed—accept it. It is not a disease, and I am sure that in due course, there will be a scientific explanation.

As Albert Einstein said, "The most beautiful and most profound religious and metaphysical emotions that we can experience are the sensations of the mystical. And this mysticality is the power of all true science."(Barnett 1957; 105)

To all cardiac transplant patients, God has blessed you with a new life, and if your new heart came with beautiful emotions (cellular memories), the more the better. Enjoy them.

THREE DAUGHTERS

Sylvia Tobin, a very pleasant seventy-five-year-old female, came to the ER with a chief complaint of chest pain. She described the pain as severe and retrosternal in location, accompanied by nausea and cold sweats. Her symptoms had started about one week before when she'd had her first episode of chest pain. She did not pay much attention to it and thought it was indigestion because the pain subsided when she took antacids. While going for her daily walk a day before admission to the hospital, she felt a quivering sensation, which she described as butterflies in her chest and difficulty in breathing. She broke out in cold sweats and felt dizzy but did not pass out. Since then, she said, her tiredness has persisted, and she has been feeling "washed out." Last night, the pain had awakened her from sleep, and she decided to come to the hospital. All of this I learned from the case history the medical resident gave me when I responded to his emergency call.

He continued, "She has a medical history of hypercholesterolemia, hypertension, but no history of smoking. On examination, she is in moderate distress and diaphoretic, with a heart rate of one hundred ten beats per minute, blood pressure one-sixty over ninety, respiratory rate of twenty breaths per minute, and oxygen saturation is normal on room air. Auscultation of the chest reveals the breathing is bronchovesicular, no crepitation or rhonchi.[4] The rhythm of the heart is regular with S4 gallop and no murmurs or rub. A chest X-ray shows clear lungs and normal cardiac silhouette. The ECG [electrocardiogram] shows a large area of myocardial ischemia. The blood tests show that cardiac enzymes are elevated, but kidney and liver functions are normal."

In summary, Sylvia was suffering from acute coronary syndrome—a spectrum of acute myocardial ischemia ranging from unstable angina pectoris to myocardial infarction. This is usually caused by an abrupt cut of the blood supply to the heart muscle by ruptured atherosclerotic plaque[28] in the coronary artery. The damage to the heart muscle is related to both the degree of atherosclerotic stenosis in the coronary artery and to the duration of sudden occlusion. If the occlusion is complete and remains for more than thirty minutes, infarction occurs.

"Please call code MI [myocardial infarction]," I instructed the resident.

It is a well-known fact that persons seventy-five years of age or older constitute 6.1 percent of the US population but account for 36 percent of acute myocardial infarction and 61 percent of deaths. The American College of Cardiology has a protocol for the treatment of acute myocardial infarction. The goal of code MI is to open the blocked vessels within ninety minutes after the patient's arrival; this minimizes the damage to the heart muscle and reduces mortality.

When taking care of a patient with acute myocardial infarction, the cardiologist's mantra, "Time Is Muscle," is the guiding principle. The primary percutaneous transluminal coronary angioplasty (PTCA) or percutaneous coronary intervention (PCI; i.e., balloon/stent)[29] is accomplished by cardiac catheterization, where a guide wire is inserted into the occluded coronary artery, and a small balloon is threaded over the guide wire and inflated in an attempt to open the blockage and restore blood flow. For treatment of acute myocardial infarction, the primary PCI is preferred over the thrombolytic (clot busters) because of lower risk of serious bleeding and strokes.

The use of primary PCI may be limited by the availability of the facilities and the personnel required to perform the procedure in a timely fashion. Sylvia was lucky to be in Robert Wood Johnson (RWJ) University Hospital because the hospital has seven catheterization labs to perform primary PCI.

When I entered the room to examine her and explain the procedure prior to her signing the consent form, I found her restless and in moderate distress due to chest pain that had not subsided after the morphine injection. She was surrounded by her three daughters.

She looked at me and with a faint smile said, "Dr. Kumar, meet my three angels." She introduced her three daughters, Susan, Laurie, and Donna.

"How's your pain on a scale of one to ten?" I asked.

"Seven. It feels like an elephant is sitting on my chest," she replied.

She was rushed to the catheterization lab for urgent revascularization with primary PCI. The cardiac catheterization showed that she was suffering from triple-vessel coronary artery disease requiring bypass surgery. She was not the patient who would have benefited from primary PCI. The chest pain subsided after the angiogram,[30] but she was at high risk of suffering a major heart attack and its associated dreaded complications of sudden cardiac death or left ventricular pump failure.

During the family meeting, I was in favor of sending Sylvia for urgent bypass surgery, but her daughters were concerned that the heart surgery was too much stress for her age; they were dead set against it. The daughters kept on repeating the same argument—that she was too old to go for heart surgery. They did not ask my opinion about the risk of surgery. They did not ask their mother how she felt about it.

This created an unpleasant situation because I strongly believe that gerontophobia[31] in medical decision making is harmful. This kind of prejudice on the part of family members has a toxic effect on the doctor's clinical evaluation. It upsets me when I see the punitive attitude of children toward their older parents, and I confront them head-on by saying, "I will not give eighteenth-century treatment to my older patients while we are living in the twenty-first century." Ironically, in eighteenth-century New England, old age was a badge of honor; it was common for people to make themselves seem older by adding years to their real age. Some people called old age the "great liberator." Older people are full of practical wisdom and don't worry what other people think. Older people don't have to prove their worth. With age, we learn what is important in life; we learn how to manage stress, anxiety, and conflicts.

We start aging the day we are born. Old age is a blessing either through genetic selection, affluence, or sheer luck. While getting old, the most important thing is to keep the "flame of curiosity" burning. Every day we live should be a new adventure and a new experience. Studies have shown that as we age, it is new experiences—not more material possessions—that keep us young and happy.

While taking care of my older patients, I always keep in mind the wise words of the British psychoanalyst D. W. Winnicott: "May I be alive when I die."(The life of D.W. Winnicott: 25)

It was not fair to Sylvia that her daughters were deciding her fate solely on the basis of her age and without her input. She was capable of deciding what was best for her; nobody knew her desires or her expectations. What was most important to *her*? What were *her* worries? The daughters talked about her age but did not say a single word about their mother's dreams. My job was to find out what Sylvia wanted—what was most important to her.

After cardiac catheterization, I knew the disease and the anatomy of her heart, but I did not know her inner core, her psyche, or her fears. I did not know her (so to speak) bucket list. These are important factors that I have to take into consideration before fighting with her daughters for her bypass surgery. The disagreement between me and her daughters prompted me to arrange a second family meeting in her room. I wanted her to participate fully in deciding her fate.

"Sylvia, the cardiac catheterization shows that you have blockage in three major vessels that supply blood to the heart muscle, and if we do not fix the blockage, I am afraid you will end up with a heart attack," I said.

"What are my options?" she asked.

"Knowing you"—I deliberately said "knowing you" in front of her daughters because I had talked to her separately and discussed things that were important and mattered—"the bypass surgery is the best option," I said.

"Tell her what can go wrong during heart surgery. She can die, have a stroke or infection, and then who will take care of her?" Susan said ungraciously.

Laurie and Donna nodded their heads in unison, indicating that they agreed with Susan. In a way, they were threatening Sylvia not to go against their wishes. Instead of supporting and helping her, they were making her anxious and miserable. I hated their behavior because for the last couple of days, I had been boosting her psyche with positive talks. I was preparing her psychologically because after major surgery, the recovery of a patient depends upon the physical disability as well as the patient's attitude toward the treatment. The patient's expectations about how he or she will do after surgery is directly proportional to his or her attitude before the surgery.

An optimistic attitude can do wonders for patient recovery. The power of positive thinking is real; the mind-body connection is real. I have seen it in my practice.

Can we force a person to have a positive attitude? Can a pessimist become an optimist?

In her book *Rethinking Positive Thinking*, Professor Gabriele Oettingen introduces us to the concept of "mental contrasting." He writes, "when people pair their optimistic dreams about the future with obstacles that prevent them from reaching that goal. Mental contrasting needs to occur in the right order; it is important to experience our dreams, and then to switch gears, to mentally face reality."

According to Professor Oettingen, rethinking positive thinking is a four-step process called WOOP: Wish, Outcome, Obstacle, and Plan.

Mrs. Tobin had all the important tools of WOOP. It was not a positive fantasy on my part to recommend heart surgery to her. I was trained as a scientist and believed in evidence-based medicine. My relationship with her was not paternalistic. Her heart was strong, and her coronary arteries were capable of surviving a bypass. She had wishes and dreams to live the rest of her life without the fear of becoming disabled. She wanted to live a meaningful life, and she was willing to take her chances and go for the surgery. On the basis of the cardiac catheterization findings, I was very optimistic about the outcome of the surgery. Her daughters' attitude was obstructive and counterproductive. It was making her depressed; she was worried. She did not want to destroy her relationship with them. She was conflicted in her mind and scared of disintegrating her social integration with family. In spite of my recommendation, her daughters were adamantly against surgery. I advised them to get a second opinion, but they refused.

Mrs. Tobin started showing signs of "elder vulnerability"—a sense of hopelessness due to the combination of poor health and crumbling social support from her daughters.

Old age can be a blessing or a hell, depending upon our social integration or isolation. The positive influence of social relationships on the recovery of a patient from a health crisis and preserving memory is well known.

The concept or theory of social integration was first described by French sociologist Émile Durkheim. In 1897 he wrote one of his most important books, *Suicide*. In it, Professor Durkheim discussed his concept of social integration. He believed that society exerted a powerful force on individuals. The suicide rate of a segment of society in Paris was directly proportional to social relationships/integration. A society that was integrated had a lower incidence of suicide rate and better mental health.

Social integration is a dynamic process that needs constant nurturing and effort. It creates a secure base from which a person can venture out and make tough decisions in life, such as the decision that Sylvia was agonizing over—whether to have or not have bypass surgery.

A global look at longevity shows us the important contribution of social integration in prolonging life. There are four geographical locations/population groups where people's life expectancy is the highest.

1. Okinawa, Japan: Women outlive men in most of the world, and Japanese women in Okinawa are among the longest-lived of all. The average life expectancy is about eighty-three years.
2. Sardinia, Italy: This island is home to some of the world's oldest people.
3. Costa Rica: The life expectancy in Costa Rica and United States is the same. However, there is a day-and-night

difference between the Costa Rican and US health-care systems.

4. Seventh-Day Adventists: The life expectancy of Adventists in the United States is about ten years longer than the rest of the population.

Although these societies are topographically and culturally different, they share four common denominators:

1. Genetics: This is the most important factor. We have no control over it, nor can we modify it.
2. Diet: The people living in the above-mentioned societies eat whatever Mother Nature gives them. They don't exploit their natural resources for the sake of profit. These people are different; they don't feel that Mother Nature is a source of wealth. They eat simple, wholesome, and fresh natural food. No chemicals or preservatives are used.
3. Spirituality: This includes a sense of connection to something bigger than us. Many spiritual traditions use contemplative practices that are associated with better health and well-being.
4. Social Integration: This is one of the most important factors for prolonging life expectancy in the Japanese and Adventists. An Okinawan grandmother is well integrated into the fabric of society. Her children and grandchildren visit her regularly, sharing meals and evening teas. She is not waiting for a Mother's Day card or reverse-charge telephone calls from children on her birthday.

Social integration, or building healthy relationships, is a slow and laborious process that needs constant nurturing with unconditional love, compassion, and loyalty. It requires a lot of effort and precious finite time that we all have on Earth.

Social isolation and disintegration can occur when an old person, who has lived all his or her life in a community, decides to leave it. He or she leaves friends, children, and grandchildren and retires in places like Florida and Las Vegas. It is beyond my comprehension how a person can bulldoze his or her social edifice and leave. I strongly discourage patients against this move. I think that it will have devastating consequences on their physical and mental health. According to a study published in *The European Heart Journal*, the lack of social integration independently predicted recurrent cardiac events. The effect of social integration on cardiovascular health is as good as running a marathon.

How can we achieve social integration? It is not difficult. It requires a new mind-set and greater effort. Go out to dinner with friends, invite them to your home, and share your blessings with them. Adapt to a new way of thinking. With adaptation, we become more open by nature, more transparent, more trustworthy, and enjoy by doing something we human beings have always been very good at—sharing.

When we live a spiritually and socially integrated life in old age, with all its inherent problems, it is still God's blessing. Called the "great liberator," old age enables us to attain serenity and savor life. Cleopatra bathed in asses' milk to stay young and beautiful but did not live long enough to find out if it worked. My sincere advice to all is this: it doesn't help to complain about your age—accept and enjoy it.

Because of her age, Sylvia was vulnerable to the wishes of her daughters. I was worried that she might change her mind and refuse to go for bypass surgery. We were wasting precious time deciding about her surgery. While she was waiting in the CCU with a bomb ticking in her chest, social workers and I were trying our best to get the daughters' permission, but their behavior continued to be pathologically obstructive. By going against the wishes of her daughters, I was afraid that Sylvia was going to destroy her relationship with them. To recover and heal from surgery, she needed all the moral as well as social support that she could get. What to do?

Next day, after seeing her, I had a long discussion with Sylvia about her daughters' objections to and my strong recommenda-tions for the surgery. I wanted her to decide. She was mentally competent to give consent, and the daughters had no legal right to deny their mother her surgery.

She stayed calm and after thinking for moment said to her daughters, "I will need your prayers, not your sympathies. I will take my chances and go for the surgery."

"Well, it's your life. Do what you like to do with it," Susan said coldly, and they left the room.

I was proud of Sylvia because she was not intimidated or bullied by her daughters. She decided to be the master of her own destiny. The daughters were of the opinion that she was too old and ready to die, but she was not ready to quit. She had a strong will and a burning desire to live. She said, "I will go when the good Lord calls me." Sadly, the daughters were disconnected from her inner core. Also, who knows what was their motive?

Finally, she went for bypass surgery. Before the operation, I met her in the preoperative room and was surprised to find out that she was alone; her daughters were not by her bedside to comfort or give moral support. I gave her a kiss and wished her good luck. Her surgery was uneventful; she had triple-vessel bypass grafts and came off the pump without inotropes.

Next day, I saw her in the Surgical Intensive Care Unit, sitting in a chair and complaining about food. Her postop recovery was miraculous. After the surgery, she was given a pillow known as a heart pillow, cough pillow, or cardiac pillow. It is a simple, wonderful tool that is utilized to lessen the pain during postop recovery. It is a perfect combination of high- and low-tech treatment. The cardiac pillow is used to splint the fracture in the sternum and provide support to the area of the chest that is healing. After heart surgery, the patient is given breathing exercises and is expected to get rid of secretions by coughing. These are extremely painful exercises when the sternum is fractured. The cardiac pillow, by splinting the fractured sternum, reduces the amount of pain patients experience when coughing, moving, or taking deep breaths.

The cardiac pillow quickly becomes patients' trusted companion. Following their full recovery, heart patients often keep their pillows around as a reminder of how far they have come; nurses and doctors write comments and draw cartoons to encourage the patient to continue living a healthy lifestyle—a celebration of a new beginning.

Sylvia's friends decorated her red-colored cardiac pillow with colorful beads from Mardi Gras and asked me to write my comment in the center of the pillow—a special honor indeed!

My comment was, "The sky is the limit—finish your bucket list." There were plenty of comments from nurses and doctors but no comments or best wishes from her three daughters.

She was transferred to cardiac rehabilitation for further recuperation.

After cardiac rehabilitation, when I saw Sylvia for a follow-up, she was the essence of sartorial splendor: hair and nails well done, a new fur coat with matching shirts, lipstick, and pants.

"The heart surgery did wonders for me," she said. She looked at Susan and continued sarcastically, "Thank God I had sense to listen to my doctors."

After complimenting her new look and fur coat, I said, "The EKG is back to normal. There is no evidence of heart damage, and I am very pleased with the postop recovery."

"The new fur coat—it is what the doctor ordered?" she asked.

"What do you mean?" I asked.

"You wrote a prescription on my cardiac pillow: 'Finish your bucket list.' Well, the fur coat was on the list." She looked at Susan with a stern and resolved face. Susan gripped the arms of the chair, not liking her mother's attitude. I was also surprised to find that after heart surgery, Sylvia's demeanor had changed. She became more assertive and feisty. Before heart surgery, she seldom expressed her opinions. Most of the time, willingly or unwillingly, she'd agreed with her daughters.

Once I asked her why she was scared of expressing herself.

"I am a *surrendered mother*," she replied. She closed her eyes and after a moment of silence continued. "The stress of facing an unpredictable future in old age forces us to surrender our feelings and desires to the wishes of children. Old age is like living in a glasshouse; there are new cracks every day, and you need someone to mend these cracks. To protect this house from crumbling, we old folks surrender, let go of our dreams, and just live in the moment." This was Sylvia's mind-set before heart surgery, and now, after heart surgery, I was seeing a new, rejuvenated person who was not scared of expressing and fulfilling her desires. It was a sea change in her demeanor, and I liked it.

"What happened to her during surgery? Did she suffer a stroke? Her behavior is completely alien to us; she is not the mother we knew. Before the heart surgery, she was cautious and very frugal, but now she is wasting money on things that she does not need," Susan said.

I was saddened to see Sylvia being humiliated and accused of wasting money. She looked at me but stayed quiet.

"If she continues to waste money, what will happen when she is old and runs out of money?" her middle daughter, Laurie, asked.

"I am already old. How long am I going to live? So let me spend some of the money I am lucky enough to have. I am quite capable of taking care of my finances," Sylvia replied with an unexpected smile.

She looked at me, deliberately ignoring her daughters as if they were not sitting next to her, and said, "My husband died young and left me with three girls. I raised them alone, working two jobs, saving, and never thinking of getting married again. I suffered but never complained. I sacrificed my youth and my dreams so that my daughters could stay safe. When I got sick and was looking for a helping hand, these girls walked out on me. Now, I don't need their advice or help." She stood up, shook my hand, and thanked me. With a resolute demeanor but a deep sadness at the core of her consciousness, she walked out of the room, leaving her daughters sitting and pondering.

"She is settling her scores with us?" Susan asked, looking at me for a response.

"Nobody is above revenge. Life is karmic balance. What goes around, comes around," I elaborated. Susan did not like my answer.

"I think that something went wrong with her brain during surgery and you are not telling us," Laurie said accusingly. They left the room threatening me with a lawsuit.

There were no signs of a stroke. The CT scan and MRI of her brain showed age-related changes in the microcirculation but no evidence of brain damage. Sylvia was enrolled in a cardiac rehabilitation program, which she completed successfully. She resurrected her friendship with a female high school classmate who became her constant companion during visits to the doctor and other social outings. She started a new life with no regrets or remorse and severed her relationships with her daughters—no mercy, no forgiveness, no reconciliation.

It is well known that anything that shatters our sense of safety tends to produce a powerful reaction. The most hateful responses are provoked when we are betrayed by loved ones. Sylvia's life was built around her daughters, and she rightfully expected their support. However, at the time of crisis when the girls did not help her, she responded with extreme vindictiveness.

What happened? Was there a connection between heart surgery and her changed personality? What poisoned Sylvia's relationships with her daughters? Was it an inappropriate emotional response, or were there some physical changes occurring in her brain? These were some troubling questions on my mind after Sylvia left the office.

During the operation, Sylvia's heart was stopped to perform bypass surgery. The oxygenated blood to the brain and the rest of her body was supplied through a special machine, the heart-lung machine. A Soviet scientist, Sergei Brukhonenko, developed the first heart-lung machine for total body perfusion in 1926. The first successful open-heart procedure on humans utilizing the heart-lung machine was performed by John Gibbon on May 6, 1953, at Thomas Jefferson University Hospital in Philadelphia. He repaired an atrial septal defect in an eighteen-year-old woman.

The heart-lung machine consists of two main functional units: the pump and the oxygenator. The venous blood from the patient is diverted to the oxygenator, and the oxygen-deprived blood is replaced by oxygen-rich blood through a series of tubes/cannulas. The oxygenated blood is pumped or transfused back through a tube/cannula inserted in the ascending aorta proximal to the origin of carotid arteries that supply blood to the brain. Microembolization,[32] especially during aortic cannulation, is the most dreaded and unpredictable complication of bypass surgery.

I think Sylvia's subtle personality changes were most likely due to a mild degree of "post–bypass surgery cognitive dysfunction." This is presumed to be due to microembolization from the heart-lung machine and aorta, thus disrupting or destroying the microcirculation to the prefrontal lobes of the brain.

The frontal lobes lie anterior in the brain; they are larger in humans (30 percent of cerebrum) than in any other primate. The most anterior part of the frontal lobes (areas 9–12 and 45–47) are sometimes referred to as the prefrontal areas. The prefrontal areas are particularly well developed in human beings and are the most mysterious part of the frontal cortex. For some, it is the seat of human intellectual and emotional capabilities. For others, it is not much more than the front bumper for the rest of the brain.

In 1964, the noted neuropsychologist Hans-Lukas Teuber described the study of the prefrontal cortex as a "riddle or an enigma" because it is inexcitable—giving no response to electrical stimuli.

The prefrontal component of the cerebral system supports goal-directed behavior. This lobe is often cited as part of the brain responsible for the ability to decide between good and bad choices and to recognize the consequences of different actions. It monitors and controls many concepts of mental activities—our thoughts and actions. It helps us to see goodness in humanity and gives us a sense of compassion and connectedness. A highly developed prefrontal brain is a blessing to us because without it, we would become two-legged, thinking monsters who have an infinite capacity to harm and kill. The prefrontal cortex civilizes our behavior and calms the animal instincts that are percolating at the subconscious level.

According to *The Principle of Neurology*, "the frontal cortex is the subject of a vast literature and endless speculation, [but] a unified concept of their function has not emerged. There is no doubt that the mind is greatly altered by disease of the frontal cortex but often difficult to say how it is changed."

There is no escape from the mysterious or, I might say, mystical nature of prefrontal brain maladies. We cardiologists see them after heart surgery but are not able to pinpoint the exact etiology.

The Vedas have elegantly expressed the mystical nature of our relationship with the universe: "As is the human body, so is the cosmic body; as is the human mind, so is the cosmic mind."

Is the prefrontal brain our connection to the cosmic brain? The answer to this question depends upon how we interpret the metaphysical nature of our existence in the universe.

It was pure conjecture or speculation that Sylvia suffered some kind of damage to the frontal cortex, but there were no tests available to confirm it—no definite answers, just speculation.

Even many years after heart surgery, Sylvia still showed no signs of dementia or deterioration of cognitive impairment, but she developed a weird sense of humor that sometimes annoyed her friends.

During an office visit one winter morning, I asked her whether she gets chest pain while exercising.

She replied with a straight face, "No, I got my nitro."

It was a confusing and ambiguous answer. Why was she using nitro pills if she had no symptoms such as chest pain or angina?

She continued, "Since I got nitro, my life has changed. I eat with nitro, sleep with nitro, and play with nitro."

I thought that Sylvia started showing early signs of Alzheimer's. I asked a few questions to test her memory. She replied appropriately.

"Nitro was also on my bucket list," she said with a mischievous chuckle.

"What do you mean?" I asked.

"I've been volunteering at an animal shelter, and last month, I adopted a beautiful Persian cat. I call her Nitro," she said.

Obviously, she had no signs of Alzheimer's. I was impressed by her selection of the cat for adoption. A Persian cat, I think, is the best companion for cardiac patients. It is quiet, placid in nature, and adapts well to apartment living. It has an abundance of unconditional love and affection for its owner and is very friendly to strangers.

I congratulated her for choosing a perfect companion and told Sylvia that I was planning to send her to a neurologist for evaluation, thinking she was getting Alzheimer's. She laughed and was proud of the fact that she was able to trick me.

Sylvia would start and finish her conversations with brief, gentle but inappropriate giggling or laughing. This is the most common manifestation of postop prefrontal cognitive impairment I have seen. The patient gives the impression of being happy all the time. There were no other signs of deterioration of her mental faculties. She was in excellent health. She had no other major illnesses except mild arthritis in both hips. She went with her friends to play bingo and continued volunteering at her church and animal shelter.

While coming out of a restaurant after celebrating her eighty-fifth birthday, she had taken a fall and broke her right hip. She was admitted in the hospital. The tests showed osteoporosis. I was consulted for pre-op cardiac clearance.

When I entered the room to examine her, she was lying flat on the stretcher, and her three daughters were sitting next to her. She was in excruciating pain but had a gentle smile with a tinge of sadness on her face. She greeted me with her usual laughs. Her daughters did not like that.

"How can she keep on giggling? She should be crying in pain, not laughing," Susan inquired.

I did not answer her. After reviewing the electrocardiogram and labs, I cleared her for the hip surgery. Unlike the cardiac surgery, the postop recovery from hip surgery was complicated with a chest infection. After staying in the hospital for one week, Sylvia was transferred to a rehabilitation center for further recuperation and physical therapy.

When I saw Sylvia a few months after her discharge from the rehabilitation center, she did not seem to be happy. The hip surgery had taken its toll on her mobility. Due to osteoporosis, the hip fracture was not healing properly. She was not able to drive and depended on her daughters. She hated it. The loss of the ability to drive and the freedom that came with it was making her depressed. She started neglecting her diet and lost weight.

"I don't know what to do," she said.

"What do you mean?" I asked.

"The heart surgery gave me the wings to fly. I was happy, very active, and thought I would live forever, but the hip fracture clipped those wings. I am bothering my daughters all the time and getting in their way," she said.

"Because of osteoporosis, the hip is healing slowly, but with a good diet and more physical therapy, eventually it will heal, and you will be able to drive. In the meantime, you can stay with one of your daughters—the three angels," I suggested.

She responded with a gentle laugh. "My angels have a wonderful final solution for my problems. After discussing matters with the lawyer, they brought me this letter to sign." She handed it to me.

The letter had two sections:

Section (a) General Power of Attorney. Mrs. Tobin hereby makes and appoints Susan, Laurie, and Donna my attorneys-in-fact to ACT in my name, place, and stead in any way which I could do, if I were personally present, to the extent and I am permitted by law to act through an agent:

There were many subsections under Section (a).

Section (b) was very disturbing and unbelievable:

(1) *Mrs. Tobin will sell her house and the money from this sale and her savings will be equally divided and given to three daughters.*

(2) *Mrs. Tobin will be allowed to spend her monthly Social Security money for personal needs.*

(3) *Mrs. Tobin will live with Susan from January to April. During these four months, Susan will take care of her. She will be with Laurie from May to August and with Donna from September to December. Mrs. Tobin's care will be the sole responsibility of the daughter with whom she is living.*

After reading the letter, I took a deep breath. I did not have the courage to look at Sylvia because I heard her sobbing.

Finally, I looked at her and saw her dabbing the tears. "I am sorry to learn that these 'kind' daughters exist on Earth and hope you will not agree to this heartless and mean proposal," I said angrily.

"Dr. Kumar, do you remember how, after my heart attack, the girls misbehaved with you?" she asked.

Without waiting to hear my answer, she continued, "When the girls were insisting that I should not go for bypass surgery, I thought they were worried about my health, but now, as I see it, the motive was to get their hands on the money. They were wishing in their hearts that I would have another heart attack and die," she said.

I agreed with her conclusion. "Sylvia, I was very suspicious of your daughters when they tried to block the surgery, solely on the basis of your age. The gerontophobia was the excuse or cover-up for their greed. Money clouded their judgment and blurred the line between right and wrong," I said.

"You're right about gerontophobia and greed." She repeated my words. She understood the motives of her daughters' proposal. In spite of age and mild cognitive impairment, her mind remained quick and sharp. Before leaving the office, she folded her hands and closed her eyes as if she were praying or thinking. I did not disturb her. After a moment of silence, she looked at me with a pensive and sad demeanor and said, "I will leave this town—out of sight is out of mind. It will be prudent to run from them rather than to fight them."

"You do not have to; you were born here and lived all your life here," I said. She did not answer back. After giving me a gentle hug, she left the office. She was gone, but the sadness and anguish of a *betrayed mother* still hung in the air. She was eighty-seven years old. Where would she go? Who would take care of her? These were some of the questions that lingered after she left the office.

I did not hear from her for a few months and thought she moved out of town, but I was pleasantly surprised when she came back for a checkup. She told me that she'd had a couple of minor falls but, thank God, did not break any bones. She had sold the house and decided to move to South Carolina.

"Why South Carolina?" I asked.

"My friend from high school fell and broke her hip. Since then, she's been having a hard time living alone. She has a lovely daughter whom I met when she came to New Jersey to take care of her mother. She is a very kind and compassionate soul and treats me just like her mother. She found an assisted-living facility for both of us near her home in South Carolina," she explained.

Sylvia continued, "As my life winds down, I want to share a few personal feelings with you. I could have kept them to myself if I had not met you and would have taken them to my grave—buried and forgotten. I am grateful to you for holding my hand and helping me all these years."

"I did my job, and I am happy that you decided to live in an assisted-living facility," I said.

She took a deep breath, closed her eyes, and after a moment of silence said, "I was trapped in a loveless marriage, like Bambi trapped in quicksand. Every push to get out pulled me back. I was planning to leave my husband, but I found out I was pregnant, and within four years I had three daughters. The final push came when my husband died and left me with three little girls. All my life I've lived in a pit full of resentment, pain, and suffering, but after heart surgery, some miracle happened that changed my life forever. The darkness and deep-seated depression disappeared. For the first time in my life, I felt I was not alone; I was part of 'something' that was more than physical. The heart surgery was a life-changing spiritual experience; it liberated me from all the fears and suffering. Thanks for recommending it." She got up, gave me a gentle hug, and left.

Sylvia died peacefully a year after moving to South Carolina.

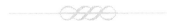

A FEW WORDS ABOUT MARRIAGE

Historian Stephanie Coontz's fascinating book, *Marriage, a History: How Love Conquered Marriage*, deals with the difficulties that human beings experience within this institution. The root cause is our expectations for marriage. According to Coontz, "People expect marriage to satisfy more of their psychological and social needs than ever before. Marriage is supposed to be free of the coercion, violence, and gender inequalities that were tolerated in the past. Individuals want marriage to meet most of their needs for intimacy and affection and all their needs for sex. Never before in history had societies thought that such a high set of expectations about marriage were either realistic or desirable. The adoption of these unprecedented goals for marriage had unanticipated and revolutionary consequences that have since come to threaten the stability of the entire institution."

In summary, in my twenty-eight years of clinical practice, the marriages I have seen can be broadly classified into three categories:

(1) "The soul-mate marriage." This marriage I truly believe is made in heaven. There is unconditional love and a sense of giving between husband and wife. This kind of marriage is not common; the relationship is built on the solid foundation of true love and kindness. The husband and wife give without expectation. They grow old sharing each other's pains and pleasures. God has blessed them with the gift of giving, and they share their blessings with children and friends. This kind of marriage will not be corrupted by the fleeting pleasures of the modern world. The husband and wife embark on a journey, and the ultimate destination is a personal and spiritual growth where there is "one soul and two bodies." I have seen this in my practice—couples married for sixty-five years and the flame of kindness and love still burning strong. The love between husband and wife emanates warm vibrations that can be felt but not seen.

(2) "The neutral/loveless marriage." In this kind of marriage, the husband and wife go through life with a give-and-take relationship. The marriage becomes a *list of expectations and regrets*. The husband and wife tolerate each other and grow old separately and die with unresolved conflicts. The quest to dominate and exploit the weakness of one's spouse is the goal of this type of marriage. The love in this marriage is a four-letter word, and it disappears like a morning fog with little heat. Life goes on without peace and happiness.

(3) "The toxic marriage." This marriage is made in hell and is one of the major risk factors to get a heart attack

or stroke. There is a taker and a loser, and the taker is a strong defender of his or her turf. The marriage is a poisonous brew of conflicts, regrets, and guilt. The taker is the winner in every exchange, and the continuous dripping of conflicts created by the taker kills the loser. A toxic marriage can be both physically and emotionally damaging. Some studies have shown as high as a 34-percent increased risk of heart disease in people who are in unhealthy relationships. A University of Copenhagen study found that those who rate their relationships as high in constant conflict are two-thirds more likely to die eleven years sooner than those who report low-conflict relationships.

I have found that patients in toxic marriages have higher rates of obesity, insulin resistance, and high blood pressure. Unhealthy relationships lead to unhealthy bodies.

Why a person would continue to live and suffer in a toxic marriage is beyond my comprehension. Is it the "side blows of karma"? The loser is paying the karmic debt for his or her past karma, and some mysterious force does not allow him or her to leave until the debt is paid. The risk of a toxic marriage causing a heart attack and killing prematurely is as strong as high cholesterol and high blood pressure. My advice is to get out of this relationship as soon as possible because the ultimate goal of the taker is to kill the loser. THIS IS THE FINAL PAYMENT OF THE KARMIC DEBT.

The case files in the next section will highlight a few of these marriages and other complex human relationships.

ALONE IN THE WORLD: FROM ORPHANAGE TO NURSING HOME

Adam, a seventy-eight-year-old white male, came to me for cardiac evaluation. He hadn't been feeling well for the last two weeks, and his wife, Rose, a patient of mine, encouraged him to see me. Rose had been coming to my office for follow-up on a regular basis, but Adam never accompanied her. Rose either came alone or with her younger sister.

Rose, at seventy-six, was very responsive to my questions. Bright-eyed Rose once told me that she did not believe in wasting words. I guess that is why my attempts to engage her in conversation in order to understand her psyche failed. After all these years of regular follow-ups, Rose's hard inner core was still a mystery to me.

Rose had bright hazel eyes, a stiff upper lip, and well-groomed blond hair. She retired as a bookkeeper, and since retirement she had been helping her church in bookkeeping. She never talked about her husband or her sister and always complimented the office staff for the good job they were doing.

However, with me, she was extremely reserved and kept her distance. This was frustrating. I felt that my treatment and evaluation were incomplete; giving her medications and not understanding her psyche for me was a job half done.

"My husband has not been feeling well; he is complaining of headache. After many days of nasty arguments, I was finally able to convince him to see you," she said.

Adam, a tall, muscular man with a round, large face and shaved head, looked like Buddha on steroids—a gentle giant. He was very liberal with his words and emotions, exactly the opposite of Rose. The Law of Attraction of Opposites Attract applied to this couple.

This concept of "opposites attract" is what we see in the behavior of subatomic particles. The positively charged particles are attracted to the negatively charged particles. In every relationship in which opposites seem to attract, we are observing two elements that are maintaining the balance between them.

In the 1950s, Robert F. Winch proposed the "opposites attract" theory, arguing that people are attracted to those whose needs conversely match their own. "A seller is always searching for a buyer."

Adam fills up what Rose lacks and vice versa. Our strengths and weaknesses not only balance us, but they also complete us.

The behavior of subatomic particles never changes, but with humans, there is a catch. Most problems in a marriage are often created by people being opposite. The things that attracted them to each other now repel them. In life, love and relationships built on one's likes and dislikes are illusions; they do not stand the test of time and evaporate at times of crisis.

Adam's history of present illness dates back about three months, when he started having mild dizzy spells. These spells were transient, usually lasting for fifteen to thirty seconds. He noticed that his dizziness was worse when he planted bushes in the garden, though he did not have any palpitation or chest pain. Before, he'd had occasional headaches; now headaches occurred daily and were of moderate intensity. Usually the pain was located in his temples and radiated to his neck. The headaches were not associated with nausea, vomiting, photophobia, or phonophobia. In the past, he'd had two episodes of double vision that were resolved after drinking cold water. He was not taking any pills and had not seen a doctor for many years.

On physical examination, he looked healthy. He had a round face, arms thicker than my legs, thighs thicker than my torso, and neck thicker than my head. Adam was a very pleasant and soft-spoken man who was retired. Before retirement he was working in a coal-mine safety department for the Mine Safety and Health Administration (MSHA).

He was lying on the bed with his eyes closed in a meditative state; there was a unique kind of calmness on his face. His pulse was 67 beats per minute and blood pressure 200/105 mmHg. His voice was normal, and his speech was fluent. His facial nerve function was normal. The neck and head examination revealed that he had a harsh carotid bruit on the left side. The rest of the physical examination and neurological examination were normal. The ECG showed mild left ventricle hypertrophy.[33]

"What is wrong with him?" Rose asked.

"He has accelerated hypertension, and if not treated, he may suffer a stroke," I said.

"Adam, when was the last time you had a blood test?" I asked.

"We've been married for the last forty years. I have never seen him go to a doctor for a checkup or blood test," Rose answered angrily.

Adam was sitting next to Rose, and he was gently tapping her hand to calm her. I saw no sign of worry on his face.

I started him on a beta-blocker and angiotensin-converting enzyme (ACE) inhibitor and asked him to get a fasting blood test, a chest X-ray, and a carotid Doppler.[34] Adam thanked me for taking care of him. Before leaving the office, he looked at me, smiled, and said, "In the past, many fires incinerated my nest, but I survived. This time, because of my age, the odds may be against me, but I'm a survivor, and I will not go down without a good fight."

Although he was gone from the office, the sadness and pain hidden in his parting words, "many fires incinerated my nest," stayed with me. I wanted to talk to him about his life and advised the nurse to give him the last appointment when he came back for follow-up. The calmness on his face and the way he responded when given the bad news of his hypertension was a reflection of strong character that was built from life struggles. He was among the rare breed of men who knew "how to collect ashes." I liked him and was looking forward to seeing him again and taking care of him.

As planned, Adam was the last patient on my schedule to see for follow-up. On examination, his blood pressure was under control: 130/80 mmHg. The review of blood tests showed high cholesterol but normal blood sugar. Carotid Doppler showed calcified plaques in both proximal internal carotid arteries (large arteries in the neck that supply blood to the brain). The echocardiogram showed mild left ventricle hypertrophy. It was obvious that he had neglected his health in spite of having both health insurance and access to doctors.

"Adam, the good news is that your blood pressure is under control, and you are out of danger of getting brain hemorrhage or stroke," I said.

"What's the bad news?" Rose asked.

"The blood test shows that the cholesterol is high, and if not treated, it gets accumulated in the arteries," I said. "There is significant accumulation of cholesterol in his carotid arteries," I elaborated.

After I stopped talking, the first thing I noticed was the abnormal eye contact—aggressive staring and anger on Rose's face. There was no sign of compassion or concern, and with a cynical smile she said, "Tell him to stop eating an omelet every morning."

"I have been eating an omelet all my life. I am not going to stop eating it now when I am seventy-eight years old," he said calmly.

It is not uncommon to hear this kind of complaint from a wife about her husband's food habits, but Rose's demeanor was hateful, aggressive, and void of compassion. I did not like it. I wanted to defend Adam, but after looking at her face, I decided to stay out of this fight.

"Please ask him how many eggs he uses for the omelet," she said.

Expectantly, I looked at Adam and found a deep sadness on his face, indicating a painful part of his life might be connected with the answer.

Suppressing his pain, he looked at me and said, "Between twelve and eighteen eggs, depending upon how hungry I am."

I was surprised to see a patient who was in relatively good health in spite of eating that many eggs daily all his life.

"The sad part is that she knows why I eat eggs, but my dear wife never misses an opportunity to bring it up," Adam said. The expression on his face was alternating between sadness and anger.

After this awkward confrontation, Adam looked at me and said, "I had a tough childhood. I grew up in an orphanage. The experience was so traumatic that the pain is still fresh in my mind. In the orphanage most of the time, I was hungry and survived on watery gruel. Every morning, supervisors ate eggs and ham for breakfast. I would hide behind the door, waiting for them to finish and praying to God that there would be left-over pieces of egg to eat. One time, I was caught for stealing a boiled egg and was whipped by the supervisor. After this incident, I promised myself that once I started earning money I would eat a lot of eggs to make that supervisor jealous in hell. Eating a big omelet for me is a cathartic event, a daily ritual—my anchor to sanity and my revenge."

"Here he goes again," Rose said, making a thoughtless, brutal, and cruel comment.

Adam did not want to discuss his diet and was eager to leave the office. I asked his wife to leave us alone so I could talk to him. She did not like it but complied.

Adam was a lonely married man. After more than forty years of marriage, there was a huge emotional deficit in his relationship with his wife. This marriage was like two stars living in separate galaxies, orbiting a predestined trajectory. There was no communication, no emotional investment, no sharing—just a lonely journey, together but separate.

People believe that marriage can insulate them from the ravages of loneliness. Such is not the case. Loneliness in marriage often happens slowly, and the disconnection one feels from his or her spouse gradually increases over time. In one study, 62.5 percent of people who reported being lonely were married and living with their partner.

Instead of discussing their mutual dreams and interests, the conversation among lonely couples becomes transactional, such as "We need milk," "Your mother called," and "Did you pay the bills?" notes Guy Winch in his book *Squeaky Wheel*.

These couples stay married because of the fear of loneliness, not knowing that the neutral, loveless marriage is going to make them lonelier. People living in this type of marriage are living in glasshouses metaphorically speaking, where new cracks of conflict, blame, and accusations appear every day. Loneliness in marriage impacts one's mental and physical health, increases the incidence of depression and heart attack, and compromises the immune system.

"Adam, how many children do you have?" I asked.

"None."

"How about brothers and sisters?"

"None. I was born prematurely, and the midwife told my mom that I would not survive the coming winter, but thank God I am still alive," he said.

I was interested to know his personal history, born as a premature baby, and how he survived winter without the help of neonatal units and incubators. He was delivered at home with no central heating or indoor plumbing.

"I was a very small baby no bigger than the size of my dad's hand. The house had no heating, but my mom was a very smart lady. She figured out how to keep me warm," he said.

"How?"

"After baking bread, she would wrap me in the blanket and put me in the warmed oven. That was my incubator. Not bad! Look at my size. Can you guess that I was a premature baby, born in a small coal-mining town, Logan, West Virginia, and lived the first six months of my life in the baking oven?"

I wanted to know more about his life in the orphanage because the emotional scars were still visible. I wanted to understand his inner core, his psyche; he would need all my help to face the ravages of disease, old age, and a lonely marriage.

What would happen if he became disabled? Who would give him a helping hand? I saw a bleak future for Adam because he was approaching the final stage of his journey. When the *last station* arrived, there would be nobody to help him get off the train.

"What happened to your parents?" I asked.

"My dad was a coal miner; he followed the footsteps of his father and grandfather and worked for a family-owned coal mine in Logan. There were no coal-mine safety laws; a canary was a miner's guide to locating the hazardous gas known as damp, possibly derived from the German word *Dampf*, which means 'steam' or 'vapor.'

"In the old days, a canary went down to work with the coal miners. The bird is a good indicator of imminent suffocation. The canary in the coal mine is always the first to go. If the canary died, the miners knew that they were soon to follow if they did not run. When the coal miners mysteriously started dying—their faces flushed and red due to carbon monoxide poisoning—canaries were used as carbon monoxide detectors," Adam said.

"Why a canary?" I asked.

"Canaries, and birds in general, are suited to this not just because they are small and portable, but because their lung anatomy makes them vulnerable to airborne poisons. The birds are great at taking in oxygen but extraordinarily sensitive to poisons in the air. A canary is taking in poison twice with each breath because of its unique respiratory system."

He took a deep breath and after a moment of silence continued, "Most of the miners die young, and the lucky ones who survived the mines end up suffering and eventually dying from chronic lung diseases such as pneumoconiosis [black lung]. The industrial revolution and economic development would not have been possible without the sacrifices of coal miners. In a mine town, the social system revolved around two kinds of occupations: coal miners and the bureaucrats who managed the coal mines. The company and mine owners owned all the stores in the town where miners can spend their money. The miners will go on strike to get more pay; the next day the company stores will increase prices, and eventually the extra money that the company gave to the miners will go back to the mine owners. The only way a miner can spend his money and not give back to the mine owners was to go out of town and spend it, but there were no roads. This is how the big wheel of capitalism revolves: give the poor workers money in one hand and take it back from the other hand. The rich and powerful people always find ways to exploit the system and win. Even today, the 'name of the game has changed but not the game.' The rich are getting richer," he said.

"What happened to your dad?" I asked.

"My dad was a hardworking, kind man. The work was dangerous and risky, but this was his only ticket to the middle class, so every week he used to do an extra shift to make more money; he wanted to get a new home and move us out of the cold shack. The supervisors would not send a canary with the miners who were doing the extra shift because the miners were easy to replace, but canaries were expensive and worth saving," he said bitterly.

"My dad and three of his buddies were on the midnight extra shift. They went into the mine without the canary. Their assignment was to open a new section of mine. Halfway through the job, they hit a large pocket of hazardous gas called black dump, which is a mixture of carbon dioxide and nitrogen. There was no canary to warn them about the early signs of hypercapnia [carbon dioxide poisoning], like headache and flushed skin. Carbon monoxide is a colorless, odorless, and tasteless gas, and once it reaches a critical level in the blood, a person becomes disoriented and dies. That is what happened to my dad and his buddies. They became confused and could not find their way back to get out of the mine, and so they died," he said.

He closed his eyes and took a deep breath. After a moment of silence, he looked up. His eyes were wet, his lips were gently twitching, and his face showed the agony and suffering of a child. He was an old man now, but still wondering and analyzing why his dad had to die to save a canary.

"My father's death crawled into my soul. Suddenly from an eight-year-old kid I became a man. I promised my mom that when I grew up I would buy her a new home. I would protect her and never leave her, but my mom didn't get to see me grow up."

"What happened to your mom?" I asked.

"Six months after Dad's death, Mom was diagnosed with ovarian cancer, and due to abdominal pain, she was bedridden most of the time. The town government and the church helped us with food. At the end of her life, my mom became very weak and was barely able to talk. However, one day she asked me to come near her, and she whispered these words in my ear: 'Adam, your pain and suffering will give you wings to fly, and remember God is your refuge, your strength, an ever-present help in trouble.' After these words, she closed her eyes and never woke up. I was nine years old and alone—no uncles or aunts to take care of me. In the town, most of the families were living in poverty and barely able to feed their kids. The town mayor, in consultation with the church, decided to put me in the orphanage."

Then he elaborated on the painful journey of going to an orphanage.

His words, "many fires incinerated my nests in the past," started making sense to me. I had plenty of pending office work to do but didn't interrupt him. Not to let him tell his life history would have been rude and painful. I think this was the first time he'd found somebody to open up his heart to, and I did not want to disappoint him. Spending time and listening to him was my ticket to get to his inner core.

He continued, "Some strange man came to the house and took me in his car to the orphanage. It took us many hours of travel. The journey seemed endless. The orphanage was a gloomy, gray building with windowless rooms. I was housed in the section of the orphanage that was reserved for 'full orphans'—children who had no living parents. Most of the kids were 'half orphans'—children who had lost a parent to death but still had one living.

"Our workday began before sunrise, when a loud clanging bell woke us up. There were no moms or dads to caress and hug us. We had fifteen minutes to get ready. Our windowless cell measured eight by five feet and was furnished with a shelf to hold books and write upon. Each room was provided with a cot and a cup filled with drinking water.

"After going to the washroom and inspection, we marched to the chapel to pray, and then spent an hour in school, learning to read, write, and do arithmetic. Breakfast lasted for half an hour, from seven to seven-thirty.

"Another bell after breakfast meant it was time to start work."

"What kind of work?" I asked.

"Generally, the boys learned and did the manufacturing jobs, while the girls learned housekeeping skills. We worked till noon, when a bell rang for dinner. The kids were not allowed to talk during meals. To communicate during meals, we used hand signals, like held up a hand for water, a thumb for vinegar. Three raised fingers meant 'bread' and one meant 'salt.'

"After meals we were required to work till five o'clock, then to wash before supper. The supper was cornmeal mush, slimy and half-cooked. Following supper, the children went back to school for two hours, and after school, there were the evening prayers and then back to our cells.

"The bell rings were the only means of communication. We were being trained like puppies to listen and follow the bell rings. There was no thinking, planning, or spontaneity for the children." He paused for a moment and looked at me.

I had nothing to say, but my demeanor must have given him the signal that I wanted to know more about this painful part of his life.

He was thankful and continued, "We were poor orphan kids but not morons. The institution treated the children as if they had no brains. Someone else was thinking for us all the time. We were living an 'artificial life,' and I was desperate to leave the orphanage."

"How did this painful chapter end?" I asked.

"God bless the US Army. My life was like going through a dark tunnel with no light in sight. After graduating from high school, I was offered a variety of jobs, but my heart was set on doing something with my life and not ending up like my dad. I heard on the radio a commercial about the army and the GI Bill, so I decided to join the army."

But there was a catch. He looked at me, and I saw this unique transformation of a sad old man into a mysteriously smiling, naughty high school kid. The fond memories of beginning a new chapter, his life in the US Army, were still shining like bright stars through gaping holes in a dark, clouded sky.

"What was the problem?" I asked curiously.

"The army only allowed eighteen-year-old draftees, and I was seventeen years old and desperate to leave the orphanage. I lied and got drafted. It was a good lie because it did not hurt anybody," he said.

The GI Bill was a godsend for kids like Adam. It started in 1944 to stimulate the economy and the education of soldiers. After the army, under the GI Bill, Adam continued his education and finally joined MSHA.

"After my dad died, I told my mom that when I grew up, I would make sure that no miner goes to work without a canary. Thank God I kept my promise," he said pensively. He closed his eyes for a moment, thanking me for listening to him.

He devoted his life to improving working conditions in the coal mines and retired from MSHA.

—⦵⦵—

A day before his birthday, Adam was admitted to the emergency room at St. Peter's University Hospital. He woke up early in the morning with an excruciating headache and fell on his way to the bathroom. When he tried to get up, he noticed weakness in his left arm and leg with slurring of speech. On neurological examination, he had left facial weakness and was not able to move his left arm and left leg. The weakness was more pronounced in his left leg than in the arm. He had mild expressive aphasia (the inability to speak). His blood pressure was 180/70, and his pulse was 80 beats per minute. He had bilateral carotid bruits; the rest of the general examination was unremarkable.

The CT scan of the head showed acute infarct[35] in the distribution of the middle cerebral artery. A carotid duplex ultrasound showed ulcerated plaques in both proximal internal carotid arteries, which was confirmed by a CT angiography.

After the examination, he was started on antihypertensive medications. I asked the physiotherapist to evaluate him for a rehabilitation program. While still in the hospital, he started showing signs of recovery. His speech improved; he was able to express himself but still had significant weakness in his left leg and was not able to ambulate independently. His wife and her sister visited him briefly but never asked the nurse about his well-being or health. They would sit in his room for half an hour and leave without talking to him. There was no sign of compassion or empathy for his illness. The cold-blooded calculations by the wife about how to deal with his sickness and not take on added responsibilities for his care were nakedly visible by her behavior. The nurses who were taking care of Adam were upset with his wife's behavior and asked me to have a family meeting to decide about rehabilitation and discharge planning.

"Adam still has a significant disability and will need help in taking care of his personal needs," I informed his wife and her sister when we had the family meeting in the hospital.

"Put him in the nursing home; we won't be able to take care of him at home," his wife said with a calculating contempt lurking in her eyes. She was a tortured soul who married Adam but never accepted him as a husband. I was not surprised to hear her response. I felt as if I were facing a crocodile rather than a human being.

"There are other options, and we should try them before sending Adam to a nursing home. I can arrange for home physiotherapy and a visiting nurse to help you and see how his disability improves," I suggested.

"My sister has very bad arthritis and needs help to move around. Her cup is full. You have to get him into a nursing home," the sister interrupted.

After the meeting, it was obvious that Adam's wife and her sister were bent upon getting rid of him and going on with their lives. Our meeting did not last long. She and her sister left the hospital without seeing him. I stayed in the room, thinking about how to tell Adam that his wife did not want him back home, and that he would end up spending the rest of his life in the nursing home.

In Hinduism, there is a concept called maya that we can loosely translate as "illusions" in English. Maya means "that which is not." According to this concept, our relationships in life are not real but illusions. Under the influence of maya, we accept the temporary as having lasting value and look for enduring relationships that don't exist. The mighty arms of time change everything, and the main cause of our unhappiness and suffering is our expectations from these illusions. We spend our lives building and nurturing relationships and have expectations. At the time of crisis, we find out that there is nothing to hold on to—no green oasis, just a mirage. It saddens us. There is nothing wrong in nurturing loving and healthy relationships with loved ones because even though these relationships are illusions, the pleasure we get from them is real. The secret of living a peaceful and contented life is to have minimal expectations from loved ones. Do kind acts and forget about them; don't have expectations for rewards or acknowledgments.

No expectations, no disappointments, and no pain.

Adam's marriage was an illusion. He was married for more than forty years, but now when he needed his wife, she walked out of his life. My job was how to lessen his pain while giving him the news that he is on his own. His pain and suffering would be directly proportional to the expectations he had from his marriage. I hoped he would accept his situation and move on. The nursing home was the last place I wanted him to go. I believed that with home physiotherapy and a little help from his wife, he would have been able to live at home.

Going to a nursing home would be a critical life experience for Adam. His going into a nursing home would be a momentous and significant event and a turning point in his life. He would lose independence, and in order to cope with these strains, he would need help from his wife, which was missing. The loss of autonomy and feeling of being powerless in the nursing home is the most stressful event to deal with for patients. The boundaries between public and private spheres in the nursing home are blurred, and patients' disabilities are on display for all strangers visiting the nursing home to see. The clear boundaries that characterize a domestic home are missing; there is no place to call home.

In the orphanage, Adam hated the fact that somebody else was making decisions for him; now as a grown-up old man, he had to accept the loss of his autonomy. I was worried that he would get depressed, and might not survive the suffocating boundaries of the nursing home, because it is well known that the life span of residents after moving into a nursing home shortens dramatically. According to a 2006 German study, 22 percent of residents die within the first six months of being put in a nursing home.

The next morning, after meeting with the social worker and the physiotherapist, I decided to inform Adam about the discharge planning. He was sitting on the reclining chair in a contemplative and pensive mood; there was a unique kind of peace on his face. All the suffering, starting from childhood up until now, did not succeed in breaking his spirit; however, I was afraid that once I told him that his wife wouldn't take him home, that he was on his own and going into a nursing home, his psyche would be shattered. He would become depressed. I was extremely careful and struggling inside to choose the words to start the conversation.

"Adam, I have good news. You are graduating from the ICU to an outpatient rehabilitation ward." My smile was feigned.

"When will I be able to go home?" he asked.

"Yesterday, I had a meeting with your wife, and she decided that the right place for you to live is the nursing home, not your own home," I said.

He looked at me but kept quiet. His color became ashen, and the peace that I observed on his face when I entered the room vanished like the morning dew on a hot summer day. The angles of his jaw started twitching, and his shoulders started shaking, indicating that he was crying. However, there were no tears in his eyes, as if he had cried so much all his life that no more tears were left to shed. His wife's refusal to help him recover from illness was the watershed event that broke his spirit, and he never recovered from it. He stopped talking, and most of the day, he was busy reading the Bible. He started eating only one meal a day. He had no friends, no family, and the only anchor he had was his faith—remembering his mother's last words: "God is your refuge, your strength, and ever-present help in times of trouble." He was like a man who saw his emotional funeral before his physical death. I knew that he had lost the will to live, and his journey to heaven started the moment he came to know that his marriage was a sham and a big illusion. This fire incinerated him and his nest. I was seeing the ashes, and the patient I knew was gone.

The next day, he was transferred to the nursing home where he started a new life, not much different than what he had when he was in the orphanage. As a child, he had no other option but to live in the orphanage. Now as an old man, who had limited time left on this earth, he had an option to live at home but was helpless. His wife had all the legal rights to decide his fate.

His wife never came to see me for her follow-up, nor did she call to let me know about Adam's health. I got busy taking care of other patients, and in the nursing home he was assigned to a different doctor.

He was readmitted to St. Peter's University Hospital with aspiration pneumonia, and the ER doctor called me to see him as soon as possible; his blood oxygen level was low, and he was refusing treatment. I rushed to the ER. When I saw Adam, I could not believe my eyes. After four months inside the nursing home, his physical condition had deteriorated with extreme loss of weight due to loss of subcutaneous fat and muscles throughout the body, as if he had been living in a concentration camp. He was in a skeletal-looking state—all skin and bones. His eye sockets were sunken. His face was thin, drawn, hopeless, and vacant.

His collar bones and ribs were sticking out and pronounced. The mouth and tongue were dry with halitosis (bad breath). He was lying in a submissive fetal position, passive and depressed. The blood chemistry showed low sodium and potassium levels, anemia, and renal failure. In summary, he was emaciated and dehydrated, a classic case of neglected personal and medical care he'd received in the nursing home.

It was a painful sight because I knew how he looked when I first met him. I used to call him Buddha on steroids. He was strong and in excellent physical health, but now nothing about his appearance looked familiar to me. The Adam I knew as a person was gone. He looked at me and closed his eyes as if saying good-bye.

Thank God he had a living will because he was hypoxic, and we were planning to put him on a respirator. After advising the nursing staff to give him oxygen and antibiotics, I went to the waiting room to talk to his wife, but there was nobody waiting for me. When I asked the unit clerk to get ahold of his wife, I was told that the transfer form from the nursing home indicated "Marital status: Divorced."

According to a joint study done by Purdue University-Indianapolis and the University of Michigan, it's a well-known fact that the divorce rate spikes among a couple if a spouse becomes sick. The risk of divorce increases when the wife becomes seriously ill, but such is not the case when the husband becomes ill. The study does not analyze why this is so, but it speculates that gender norms around caregiving play a factor. The wife is used to being the caregiver, and when she gets sick and can't be the caregiver, the gender norm changes, which sets the stage for divorce. A marriage that has been nurtured with love, compassion, and the gift of giving will survive this personal seismic event. It is the toxic or the loveless marriage that crumbles when the gender norm changes. Adam's wife was not a caregiver type. She divorced him and with her sister moved to Florida.

In spite of multiple antibiotics and oxygen treatment, there was no significant change in his breathing difficulty, and he died peacefully without intubation or respirator. I could not say good-bye to him because he died suddenly in cardiac arrest. The unit nurse handed me a letter from Adam thanking the nurses and doctors for taking care of him. His last words were, "My ride was lonely, but thank God I am finishing this wonderful journey without regrets." He died on his eighty-first birthday.

He wanted to give a gift to his nurse for her kind and compassionate care, but there was nobody, no relatives whom he could request to get a box of chocolates or cookies. He left his most precious possession that was a source of his strength for her—his family's Bible. Glued to the back cover of the Bible, we found the following 1845 poem by Elizabeth Barrett Browning:

A Thought for a Lonely Deathbed

If God compel thee to this destiny,
To die alone, with none beside thy bed
To ruffle round with sobs thy last word said
And mark with tears the pulses ebb from thee—
Pray then alone—"O Christ, come tenderly!
By thy forsaken Sonship—and the red.
Dear wine-press—and the wilderness outspread—
And the lone garden where thine agony
Fell bloody from thy brow—by all of those
Permitted desolations, comfort mine!
No earthly friend being near me, interpose
No deathly angel 'twixt my face and Thine,
But stop Thyself to gather my life's rose,
And smile away my mortal to Divine!"

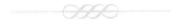

THE PATIENT WITH SLOT-MACHINE SYNDROME AND HIS SOUL MATE

The development of a disease in a patient has two well-known components:

* Genetic component
* Environmental components

A true monogenic genetic disorder[36] will cause the disease regardless of the environmental factors. The fate of a person who is carrying a monogenic genetic disorder is sealed the day he or she is born. The modifications of environmental risk factors play a minor role in the final outcome; they may postpone the true manifestation of the disease, but eventually the genetic disorder prevails and kills the patient. In the majority of cases, though, the burden of the *genetic cross* that a person is born to carry can be reduced by modifying the risk factors.

A less recognized component in the development of disease is the arrival of a new industry. The industrial injuries may mimic the classical signs and symptoms of a common disease. The arrival of a new industry can change the environment, and these changes can affect the health and well-being of the community. The environmental impact of a new industry will bring a new set of medical problems that the community doctors have not seen. The major role of environmental factors in causing a disease should change our focus. Instead of spending time and money on treating the disease, the focus of intervention must shift from the individual to the environment. To make a meaningful difference in the health of a community, we must provide a healthy environment and modify the reaction of individuals to their environment because an "unhealthy environment will produce an unhealthy community."

How do we balance the economic well-being of a community with a healthy environment? This can be achieved by proper education and modification of behavior of individuals to the changing environment.

We can compare a sickness or disease to a "black box." The monogenic genetic component puts a patient right in the middle of the box, and the modification of environmental factors will not help these patients escape the box. The vast majority of patients are at the margins of the box, either inside or outside, depending on their genetics, and in these patients the modification of risk factors plays a critical role in deciding between sickness and health. The patients who are genetically predisposed to heart disease can improve their health by modifying risk factors such as diet, exercise, and reducing mental and physical stress. On the other hand, even with healthy genes, a person can get heart disease by living or working in an unhealthy environment.

THE ROLE OF ATLANTIC CITY IN CARDIAC HEALTH

Before the birth of the casino industry, Atlantic City had a colorful history. The location of a city hugging the ocean was ideal to develop it as a resort city and to bring people in large numbers. Direct train service was established in 1874; more than five hundred thousand people came to this resort town every year. There were no cars or superhighways. Coming to Atlantic City by train and enjoying the ocean became very popular. The growing popularity of Atlantic City and the need to accommodate more visitors led to the establishment of a second railroad line in 1878 between Philadelphia and Atlantic City.

During the early part of the twentieth century, Atlantic City was a booming town. The popular candy, saltwater taffy, was conceived of in Atlantic City. The story is that a candy store got flooded after a fierce storm, soaking the taffy with salty Atlantic Ocean water. The store sold these "ruined" candies as "Salt-Water Taffy." Kids loved them, and so saltwater taffy was born.

The decline of Atlantic City began in the mid-twentieth century, after World War II. The city was plagued with crime and corruption. The general economic decline affected Atlantic City as well as most of the East Coast cities. There were multiple reasons for the resort's decline.

Automobiles became readily available to Americans after the war. This allowed people to come and go as they pleased, and instead of spending weeks at a resort city, they stayed for only a day or two.

The advent of suburbia allowed many families to move into private houses with all the luxuries of a resort's amenities, such as air conditioning and swimming pools. This diminished people's interest in going to beach resorts in the hot summer.

Cheap jet service to other premier resorts in Florida and the Caribbean Islands would further diminish Atlantic City's appeal.

In an effort to revitalize the city, in 1976 New Jersey voters approved casino gambling for Atlantic City. The arrival and popularity of the casino industry would change the eating habits of my patients. They started flocking to Atlantic City in droves. The toxic brew of gambling and eating cheap, unhealthy buffet food created a whole new set of medical problems.

CASE FILE

Walter was a seventy-year-old white male who came to my office with a complaint of chest discomfort/pain. He described the pain as a dull ache that had been radiating to his right arm. The pain did not change when walking but got worse when taking deep breaths.

He had no history of heart disease and had not seen a doctor for many years. He said he "hates taking pills." He did not smoke but drank socially.

Walter was a stocky man of medium height with a gentle smile, penetrating light-blue eyes, and a receding hairline with short blond hair. A man of few words, he was very short and to the point in answering my questions. There was a reassuring kind of calmness in his demeanor. There was no sign of anxiety or nervousness as he lay on the examination bed with his eyes closed in a meditative state while waiting for further evaluation.

On examination, he appeared uncomfortable when I asked him to "take a deep breath." His heart rate was 100 beats per minute, his blood pressure was 190/105 mmHg, his respiratory rate was 21 beats per minutes, and he had an oxygen saturation of 98 percent on room air.

There was a large area of ecchymosis (bruise) on the medial (inner) side of his right upper arm, and it was tender to the touch. An auscultation of the neck revealed left carotid bruit; a chest examination was unremarkable; and the lung fields were clear. There was a regular sinus rhythm with prominent S4 gallop and grade 2/6 ejection systolic murmur in the aortic area. The electrocardiogram showed normal sinus rhythm with mild left ventricle hypertrophy.

After finishing the examination, I said, "Come to the consultation room, and please bring your wife." He looked at me and wondered why I wanted to talk to his wife.

The evaluation of a patient with chest pain is not complete without input from his wife, as men tend to downplay their symptoms. The accurate history of a patent's symptoms is the most important diagnostic test for the evaluation of chest pain.

The presence of his wife in the room was reassuring because I knew that she would keep him honest.

The interaction of the patient and his wife during the intake history also gives me input regarding the dynamics of their relationship, which, as I mentioned before, is as important as the other high-tech tests for the diagnosis.

The long journey of diagnosis and treatment starts with the intake history in the consultation room. It helps me to understand the "inner core" of a patient. The history and physical examination have taken a backseat in the evaluation of patients. The "high-tech but no emotional approach" to patient care is fundamentally changing the role of a doctor. I hope the *art of medicine* will not degenerate into a scenario in which the *iDoctors* sitting in front of computers are providing care to *iPatients* and forgetting that the patient's pain and suffering are real. The doctor's bill looks like an invoice from a hardware store.

The technology-driven approach to every symptom reflects our fears of being wrong; it reflects a lack of confidence in our knowledge of medicine. Doctors are becoming skilled technicians, and something precious in a doctor's calling is being lost.

After exchanging pleasantries with Walter's wife, I asked how long they had been married.

"We celebrated our fiftieth anniversary last month," she said.

Dolores was a slightly overweight woman of average height. She had a round face and a prominent nose with thick, broad-rimmed bifocal glasses. She had mildly scarred facial skin and a kind and friendly smile.

She held Walter's hand and pressed it gently to assure him that he would be all right.

"We were kids when we got married, and our friends and families predicted that the 'marriage will be over before sunset,'" she said.

Walter looked at her and remained silent, but his eyes gave it away. He was thankful to her for being kind and compassionate after fifty years of marriage. In their eyes I saw the fire, a fire that was ignited by true love still burning strong. The eyes are frequently called the "windows to the soul" and they never lie. This nonverbal language of the eyes is extremely subtle; we in the medical profession will not be able to master it if our eyes are glued to the computer screen while taking the history of a patient's illness. A true love with kindness and compassion does not need verbal validation.

After graduation from high school, Walter joined the US Navy as a sailor, and one year later he was selected to join the Navy SEALS, specializing in underwater demolition missions. "I blew up lots of Commie bridges in the Korean War," he said.

After the war, Walter came back and joined DuPont, from which he retired as a machinist. He was proud of his service to the nation and of being a SEAL. "Our SEAL unit was a unit of lions, led by lions," he said.

"Walter, how long have you been having chest pain?" I asked.

"My chest has been hurting for the last two days," he replied.

"Have you been working in the yard, planting bushes, or doing heavy lifting?" I asked.

"No."

He had no history of falls or other injuries. He looked at me expectantly, waiting for the answers and the diagnosis.

"What's wrong with my husband? Is he having a heart attack?" his wife asked.

I looked at her husband. His physical examination and history matched that of three other patients I had seen in the last month. All these patients were elderly with poor muscle mass due to lack of exercise, aside from playing slot machines and engaging in similar sedentary activities.

The classic old-style slot-machine design works on an elaborate configuration of gears and levers. A breaking system brings the spinning reels to a stop. By the nature of its design, when the mechanical slot machine is played for a long time, it exposes arm muscles to repeated microinjuries. In elderly patients with poor muscle mass, these can cause rupture or dislocation of minor muscle from its insertion point.

Chest pain is one of many causes of a heart attack. The fear of suffering a heart attack brings patients to the doctor's office, but most of the patients who walk in are not having a major cardiac event. In these patients, the etiology of chest pain is extra cardiac-like musculoskeletal or pulmonary conditions. The physical examination and proper history will further differentiate the diagnosis.

"Walter, do you go to Atlantic City?" I asked.

He was surprised to hear this question and hesitated in answering.

"He loves to go to casinos and plays the slot machines for hours," his wife said.

I saw that Walter was getting anxious. He said, "What does Atlantic City have to do with the chest pain?"

"Are you spending a lot of time playing slot machines?" I asked.

He looked at his wife, turned around, and defended his visits by replying, "The slot machine is a God-sent gift to us elderly folks. In Atlantic City, my aches, pains, and fear of getting old and not being able to take care of things disappears.

A small part of me is rejuvenated, like newly planted corn," he elaborated.

"Walter, you are suffering from 'slot-machine syndrome,'" I said.

"What is slot-machine syndrome?" his wife asked.

While you won't find this in medical textbooks, slot-machine syndrome is based on my personal observations. (My medical letter describing this syndrome was published in the *Journal of the Medical Society of New Jersey* some decades ago.) "A syndrome is a group of symptoms and signs, which, when considered together, characterize a disease," I replied. "After playing the slot machine for hours, you ruptured one of the inner muscles of your right arm and have a large hematoma [collection of blood] that was creeping toward the chest wall."

"The irony of the situation is that blowing up bridges in the Korean War was less dangerous than pulling the slot-machine handle," this proud vet said bitterly.

"What is the next step? Can you take care of him? I hope that he won't be admitted to the hospital," his wife said.

"The hematoma will resolve itself without intervention. Walter has to abstain from playing the slot machines. His arm needs rest to heal," I said.

Although Walter's chest pain was due to muscle injuries, the cardiovascular examination revealed that he had significant atherosclerosis. He was suffering from high blood pressure and a bruit in the left carotid arterial system. He was not aware of his blood cholesterol or blood sugar.

It is unfortunate to see patients like him who, in spite of health insurance, are walking around with medical problems, which, if not managed properly, could cause lifetime disabilities or death. Walter would need further evaluation by imaging studies such as a carotid Doppler, echocardiogram, and blood tests. I started him on an antihypertensive and analgesics and advised him to see me in two weeks.

Walter was not happy with the diagnosis or the low-tech treatment I recommended, such as cold compresses for the hematoma, a pain-killer, and not playing slot machines.

He looked at me in disbelief. "I came with one medical problem, and now I'm leaving this office with three." His wife appeared to be upset and angry about his bad behavior but stayed quiet.

How patients will behave with a doctor during their first visit is difficult to predict. Patients are scared of the diagnosis and worry that the disease may rob them of their dignity and self-respect and end up making them give up the things they love to do.

For doctors to earn patients' respect, it is important to trust patients with medical facts. Patients, regardless of their education or economic background, are capable of making sound decisions about their treatment options.

Walter was a proud Navy SEAL; it was difficult for him to accept the fact that the slot machine would disable and humble him. I understood his psyche and assured his wife that I was not offended.

During the follow-up visit, I found Walter more trusting and deferential. He greeted me with a classic marine salute, but it is not appropriate for a marine in civilian clothes to initiate a salute. He was a retired marine, and the salute was his way of showing gratitude and respect. The hematoma in the right arm and chest pain were resolved.

The laboratory and imaging studies showed that he had high cholesterol, nonobstructive multiple calcified plaques (cholesterol deposits) in both carotid arteries, and mildly calcified aortic valve leaflets. Walter had a time bomb ticking in his chest; he was at high risk of suffering a stroke or heart attack. The cholesterol deposits in the carotid arteries were calcified, indicating that even with aggressive cholesterol-lowering drugs he was predisposed to getting a stroke.

After a long discussion with husband and wife, I started him on cholesterol-lowering drugs, aspirin, and a low-cholesterol diet which he hated.

"I'm going to miss the casino's buffet," he said.

Dolores looked at him, shook her head, and said, "You have finished your quota of hamburgers. No more junk food in the house."

I advised him to come every three months for follow-up and continue taking his medications. She assured me that she would watch his diet. In the meantime, Dolores also became my patient.

"Dr. Kumar, Walter is on line two, and he says it is an emergency." The secretary relayed this message on the intercom.

I picked up the phone. "Walter? Dr. Kumar here."

"When Dolores stood up to sing a hymn after services, she fainted and fell to the floor. The ambulance is taking her to the hospital," he said.

After examination, the ER physician called me and gave a brief summary of clinical findings. On examination she was alert, her heart rate was regular at 32 beats per minute, and her blood pressure was 115/72, which dropped to 70/50 when she stood. She had blunt injuries, like contusions on her face, right arm, and right chest, but no focal neurological deficit.[37]

I interrupted my office schedule and rushed to the ER. On the way, I called the resident to arrange for an external pacemaker and for her to be given fluid.

I was relieved to see that she was awake and holding her husband's hand and talking to the nurse, who was busy starting the intravenous fluid.

The laboratory examination showed normal thyroid function and electrolyte level, with no evidence of a heart attack on blood examination. Her medical history was essentially unremarkable except for mild arthritis in the right knee for which she took Motrin®.

The ECG (electrocardiogram) showed bradycardia, with third-degree atrioventricular (heart) block. Dolores was suffering from a serious heart problem known as "sick sinus syndrome." The sinus node is an intrinsic pacemaker in the heart, and its function is to keep the heart beating by generating electrical impulses. When the sinus node is unable to adequately perform its function, the patient's heart rate drops. This can cause stroke, heart attack, or death.

We rushed her to the cardiac catheterization laboratory and inserted a pacemaker to bring her heart rate and blood pressure to safe levels. After the procedure she was transferred to the Cardiac Care Unit (CCU) for further recuperation and cardiac monitoring.

The overall mortality rate in patients with sick sinus, even after pacemaker insertion, continues to be high. The sick sinus is always associated with serious cardiac or other diseases. The long-term prognosis of these patients is dismal.

The next morning, I found her sitting up in a chair with the sun shining on her face. A routine examination revealed that Dolores had an artificial left eye, and her facial skin was riddled with small star-shaped scars.

She looked at me and anticipated the questions on my mind.

"Dr. Kumar, please sit down. It is a long and painful story I want to tell you," she said. "After graduating from high school, I went to nursing school because my grandmother, whom I loved the most, was bedridden from a stroke. I wanted to take care of her, and becoming a nurse was the right thing to do. When I received the acceptance letter from the nursing school, my grandmother asked my dad and my mom to take me to church and have the letter blessed by the priest. For my grandmother, nursing was God's calling, a vocation.

"I was good with books and studied hard with a well-defined mission to be the best nurse and graduated with flying colors. After graduation while working in the hospital, I developed horrible acne on my face. The acne papules were sprouting like toadstools in a forest after heavy rain, and within three months both sides of my face were covered with acne.

"I was terrified and scared because there was no treatment available for acne, like antibiotics or cosmetic surgery. The nurses were not allowed to come to work with makeup, and that prevented me from hiding the acne scars.

"Some events in life leave permanent scars; they never heal, and you carry them the rest of your life and eventually they are buried with you. I remember the day that changed my life forever. We should enjoy the present because who knows what is waiting around the corner," she said.

She looked at me and took a deep breath, as if she were preparing herself to dive into an abyss where she would revisit those monsters that had been lying dormant for a long time.

She continued, "It was a crisp, wintry day, and I was assigned to the evening shift." She shut her eyes to refresh the painful memories.

"In the middle of our rounds, the head nurse informed me that Dr. Clark (the head of the medical department) wanted to see me. Dr. Clark was a tall man with a ruddy face and crew-cut hair who retired from the army before joining the hospital. His self-appointed mission was to bring army-style discipline to the medical department. All the nurses were scared of him, and I knew that I was in trouble."

Dolores looked at me. She took off her glasses and wiped the tears from her good eye.

"'Nurse, you are not going to take care of patients,' Dr. Clark said.

"'Why not?' I asked.

"'Acne is not a pleasant thing for the sick patients to see,' Dr. Clark said. Then he said, 'There is a new treatment for acne, and I will advise that you should try it before I let you go back to patients' care.'

"I was humiliated and hurt but relieved to know that there was treatment for acne.

"'The hospital bought a new radiation-therapy machine that cures most skin diseases. The papules will disappear in ten days of radiation therapy, and in the meantime, you will be doing desk jobs,' Dr. Clark said and left the office abruptly.

"The head nurse held my hand and said, 'I have already talked to the head of radiation therapy, and he has agreed to see you in the morning.'"

The history of the use of radiation therapy for skin lesions started soon after the discovery of the X-ray in 1895. It was used to treat all kinds of skin diseases like lupus, epitheliomas, acne, and even epilepsy.

"The X-ray apparatus used for my acne had a tube and perforated sheet of metal that was securely fashioned to my face with adhesive tape," Dolores continued.

"The doctors were ignorant about calibration and the radiation doses. The therapy made me tired, and I lost my appetite. As the treatment progressed, my skin became more sensitive and irritated. The acne lesions started changing to small blisters, and eventually they would peel off like snowflakes," she said.

"The acne lesions disappeared after two weeks of radiation therapy." She paused for a moment and looked at me. "I went back to nursing care, but the fire that had been burning inside my heart to be the best nurse was gone. The way Dr. Clark humiliated and insulted me left more scars than you see on my face," she said.

"I got married, and when my daughter was in high school, I started having blurred vision in the left eye, which was diagnosed as ocular cancer [melanoma]. The left eye was removed; thank God the cancer did not spread to the brain.

"We are all born to carry the cross, but mine was a little too heavy. I went to church and asked for His forgiveness and resigned from nursing," she said.

"History has a tendency to repeat itself. Humankind has been making statements through its women since the Middle Ages," she said.

"I was the girl who brought dishonor to Dr. Clark and his medical department; to protect it, he almost killed me. Honor killing is still going on in the world; thousands of innocent girls are being killed to protect men's honor. As an Amnesty International statement says, 'The regime of honor is unforgiving; women on whom suspicion has fallen are not given the opportunity to defend themselves.' Men have no socially acceptable alternative but to remove the perceived stains on their honor by attacking and sometimes killing women either physically or emotionally, like Dr. Clark did to me," she said.

Honor killings have been around since ancient times. I remember "The Story of Ramayana." Sita, the wife of Lord Rama, was abducted by the demon king, Ravana. She was held captive for many years on the island of Lanka where Ravana unsuccessfully tried to persuade her to marry him. Lord Rama, aided by his brother Lakshan and mightly monkey general Hanuman rescued Sita.

After Lord Rama and Sita returned to Ayodhya, the citizen of his kingdom questioned the chastity of Sita during her period of capture by Ravana. To protect the honor of Lord Rama and prove her purity, Sita had to go through trial of fire. Mother Earth took her back, and she never returned.

The humiliation and pain suffered through the years by Dolores is not much different than what is being experienced by millions of women all over the world. I was relieved when Dolores stopped talking; the painful incidents in her life not just opened the old wounds but also perhaps revealed wounds she did not know she had. She was discharged from the hospital after recuperation from pacemaker surgery.

Walter was admitted because of an acute onset weakness in his right arm and difficulty speaking. The neurological symptoms started more than three hours before his admission to the emergency room. It was too late to treat him with a thrombolytic agent[38] to dissolve the blood clot in the carotid artery.

The noncontrast computerized tomography (CT) of the brain showed a large-size nonhemorrhagic stroke in the middle cerebral artery territory. The transesophageal echocardiography (TEE) showed a large, round hanging atheroma (a glob of cholesterol) with multiple atherosclerotic plaques in the arch of the ascending aorta. He was transferred to the critical care unit for further observation and treatment.

The three-hour window is the most critical factor for the prognosis of patients with stroke. The patients who come to the hospital in time—within three hours, and get treated properly, have an excellent prognosis and recover fully. The unusual delay in treatment of stroke will have devastating consequences for the patient and his or her family. After surviving a stroke, the patient may end up spending the rest of his or her life in a nursing home. The emotional impact of stroke can be just as devastating as its physical effects. The doctor who takes care of the patient is not immune from it.

The focal neurologic symptoms produced by stroke showed no improvement. Walter's general medical condition continued to deteriorate. The corner of his mouth drooped with flattening of the right nasolabial folds; he was not able to fully elevate his eyebrows. There was a slight diminishment of alertness (consciousness) and further deterioration of speech. He was unable to express his thoughts but understood verbal commands. His respiration was slightly shallow.

I met Dolores and their daughter in the family conference room to discuss his medical condition and answer the questions they had about his treatment and prognosis.

"How is my dad doing?"

"There is slight worsening of his neurologic status. He started showing early signs of brain stem compression," I said.

"What is brain stem compression?" Dolores asked.

"The massive stroke that Walter suffered is causing swelling of the brain tissues and increasing pressure inside the skull, which makes the brain tissues move from their usual position. I have already started him on steroids and hope this will reduce the brain swelling," I said.

"Dr. Kumar, you know him well. He was a Navy SEAL, and in his life, he has confronted death many times and survived. I have a bad feeling that this time he won't be able to make it. I want him to die with dignity and not to be humiliated with tubes and respirators. More than machinery, he needs humanity and compassion," she said. Dolores got up and gave me a gentle hug and said that she would like to see him.

Walter's neurologic status showed no sign of improvement; there was further deterioration of consciousness. A repeat CT scan of his brain showed multiple areas of damage that were not seen before. The hanging atheromas in the arch of aorta were the source of repeated embolization to the brain. He became unconscious and died peacefully, his wife and daughter holding his hand and the priest giving the Sacrament of the Anointing of the Sick.

In a way, Walter was a lucky man. When the last station came, he got off the train without heavy baggage: no respirator, no Foley catheter, no feeding tube—just a simple and beautiful *bon voyage*.

"It's been more than two years since Walter died, and I am still upset," Dolores said during one of her follow-up visits to the office.

"The pain and trauma never go away completely, but time is a great healer, and it always softens the pain. It chisels away the rough edges of trauma and makes it bearable, but a soft ache always stays in our hearts," I responded. There was a palpable sense of relief as she considered my comments.

"I shouldn't feel guilty that it's still hurting and I am not over it?" she asked.

"No. I think you should give yourself a break. Trauma is part of living, and it happens to all of us. Nobody is immune. It is unrealistic to expect that life will be free of suffering, pain, and disappointment. Our lives stay in a state of organized instability, and we should be conscious of the fact that sickness and death are waiting around the corner. Our lives are loaded with either posttraumatic stress or pretraumatic stress, like worrying about old age, accidents, illness, separation, and loss. We are all born into suffering."

"Like a dog without a bone, into this life we are thrown," as the music group The Doors sang.

I continued, "We all must experience pain and loss. This is the Buddhist view on suffering. The major cause of suffering is our expectation that the people we love will stay with us forever.

"This is an illusion, because the thing that does not change with the passage of time is 'the change,'" I concluded.

Accepting mortality has become harder because death is now uncommon. Over the last fifty years, medical sciences have evolved rapidly, and we have become immune to death. New technologies and advances in medical treatment are making us less comfortable with death.

Before heart surgeries, angioplasties, chemotherapies, and antibiotics, people often died when they got sick. Some people think that death is an option, a taboo, and it should stay in the closet.

The Swiss American psychiatrist Elisabeth Kübler-Ross brought death out of the closet with the publication of her book *On Death and Dying* in 1969.

When faced with the trauma of impending death, a person goes through a series of emotional stages. Kübler-Ross outlines these stages of grief and introduces the "Five Stages of Grief," known by the acronym DABDA:

1. Denial—"I am fine. This cannot be happening; it's not me." Denial is usually only a temporary defense. It stays for a short while.

2. Anger—"Why me? It's not fair. How can this happen to me and who is to blame?" This stage of grief is no stranger to doctors because we live in a culture where acceptance of death has become an alien concept. How to deal with it? Be nonjudgmental when dealing with a patient who is experiencing anger. The lack of curriculum in medical schools has poorly prepared doctors in addressing the subject of death and dying. We should be proactive and prepare loved ones to accept death as part of living.

3. Bargaining—"I would do anything for a few more years." People facing less-serious trauma can bargain and compromise, but in a matter of life and death, this does not help.

4. Depression—"I am going to die soon, so what is the point? Why bother with anything?" This stage comes when the patient has begun to accept the situation.

5. Acceptance—"I cannot fight it; I might as well prepare for it." Life is a journey, and eventually we all have to get off at the last station. I hope when the time comes, our final and last disembarkation will be peaceful and painless. Those who are dying can enter this stage of trauma much sooner than the ones they will leave behind.

Walter accepted his mortality the day he suffered massive stroke, but it took many years for Dolores to accept it.

As we know, grief is not the same for everybody, and I believe that people's response to major trauma is modulated by their cultural background. It is our faith that prepares us to collect ashes in life, and people who have no faith generally find it hard to deal with major trauma. The best way to deal with grief is not to ignore it but to lean into it. There is no definite timetable for mourning.

The willingness to accept sufferings is our key to living a spiritual and meaningful life.

Taking care of patients who are facing impending death is a difficult task for doctors. Doctors are trained to save lives, so a patient's death becomes a personal loss and defeat. It should not be that way, though; our job is to lengthen the time that stands between good health and death.

Major trauma and grief should be time for reflection and acceptance, like the hymn "Abide with Me," written by Henry Francis Lyte in 1847. He was dying from tuberculosis and survived only three weeks after its completion.

The hymn is a prayer for God to remain present with the speaker throughout life, through tribulations and trials, and through death:

Abide with me; fast falls the eventide;
The darkness deepens; Lord with me abide;
When other helpers fail and comforts flee,
Help of the helpless, O abide with me.

Swift to its close ebbs out life's little day;
Earth's joy grows dim; its glories pass away;
Change and decay in all around I see;
O Thou who changes not, abide with me.

Not a brief glance I beg, a passing word,
But as Thou dwell'st with thy disciples, Lord,
Familiar, condescending, patient, free.
Come not to sojourn, but abide with me.

Come not in terrors, as the king of kings,
But kind and good, with healings in Thy wings;
Tears for all woes, a heart for every plea.
Come, Friends of sinners, though abide with me.

Thou on my head in early youth didst smile,
And though rebellious and perverse meanwhile,
Thou have not left me, oft as I left Thee.
On to the close, O Lord, abide with me.

I need Thy presence every passing hour,
What but Thy grace can foil the tempter's powers?
Who, like Thyself, my guide and stay can be?
Through cloud and sunshine, Lord, abide with me.

I fear no foe, with Thee at hand to bless;
Ills have no weight, and tears no bitterness.
Where is death's sting? Where, grave, thy victory?
I triumph still, if Thou abide with me.

Hold Thou Thy cross before closing eyes;
Shine me through the gloom and point me to the skies;
Heaven's morning breaks, and earth's vain shadows flee;
In life, in death, O Lord, abide with me.

This hymn was a favorite of Mahatma Gandhi. It is also played by the combined band of the Indian Armed Forces during the annual Beating Retreat Ceremony held on January 29 at Vijay Chowk, New Delhi, that officially marks the end of the Republic Day celebrations.

After a certain age, we should see death as a triumph worth celebrating, not a failure.

In the Victorian period, people had a fascination with death. Instead of fearing the process of dying, they felt reverence. According to them, these were stages in the life of a beloved body and should be treasured. An entire industry grew up around the culture of mourning—special clothes, stationery, and so on.

Josephine Elizabeth Butler (April 13, 1828–December 30, 1906) was a Victorian-era British reformer and social worker. Her only daughter, Eva, died in 1863, following a fall from the stairs at their home. Mrs. Butler saw something radiant in her daughter's eyes, perhaps a reflection of God. She said, "Some glory approaching bore the reflection of that which she saw. It was as if she said, 'Now I see God.'" Death was accepted as a natural part of life.

Dolores continued, "All my life, Walter sheltered me from the pain and aggravation of modern living, but since his death, I am lost. I never bothered to ask him about our investments and insurance policies because in my heart I believed and also wished that the good Lord would take me before him. He was the only man in my life, a devoted father and a faithful husband. Three principles guided his life: country, faith, and family."

Dolores reminisced about the good life she'd had when she came to see me for a follow-up visit.

I knew Walter; he was a decent family man who loved his wife. I had fond memories of him telling me how, during the Korean War, he blew up bridges.

"The good memories help us to keep our sanity; they are stored in deeper recesses of the brain. These memories may fade over time but never go away. These are the anchors that hold us when life forces us to face major traumas," I said.

"It is almost four years since Walter passed away. My cousin and my daughter helped me to straighten out the legal problems, and thank God I am able to be on my own now. I learned how to get money from the cash machines, I got my driver's license, and every Wednesday I go with my friends to play bingo," she said.

"I am glad to know that you are getting over your grief," I said.

"I met someone named Jay at one of these bingo parties, and he asked me out on a date. I said no. He called me a couple of times. I heard from my friends that he has a reputation for being aggressive and won't take no for an answer. He was very persistent, and finally I went out with him."

"How long have you been dating him?" I asked.

"Nine months. It took me almost three months before I decided to spend a night at his house. I had mixed feelings about it, at times feeling guilty that the sanctity of the relationship I had with my husband was violated that night," she said.

"How do you feel now?" I asked.

"I was raised as a Catholic and always believed that sex is only morally exercised within the bond of marriage," she replied.

"How does Jay feel about it? Is he also Catholic?" I asked.

"Yes, he is Catholic but does not respect my feelings; he says the bitter divorce from his wife changed him forever," she explained. "Dr. Kumar, Walter respected and loved you as his doctor, and I'm glad he didn't suffer but passed away peacefully. You are more than a doctor to me; I see you as my brother, my son, my father."

"Thanks," I said.

"Jay came up with a proposal; he says that if I agree to it, this will take our relationship forward to a deeper level. I feel uncomfortable discussing this with my daughter," she stated.

"What kind of proposal?" I inquired.

"He advised me to sell my house and move into his house. That way, he says, we can spend more time together, get to know each other better, and hopefully get married one day," she explained.

"What was your response?" I queried.

"Since then, I have been confused and scared. I don't want to lose him. After Walter died, I felt lonely and needed company, but to sell the house and move in with him does not feel right. It is also against the tenets of my faith, as a Catholic Christian, to live with this man who is not my husband. What should I do?" she asked.

"You should not sell the house because if he breaks off the relationship and leaves, where are you going to stay?"

She looked at me but remained silent.

I advised her, "Tell him that he should sell his house and move into your house. Dolores, since you consider me more than your cardiologist, I will advise you to discuss this matter with your daughter, especially if you decide to sell the house. This world is full of scoundrels, and I hope Jay is not one of them," I warned her.

"We're going out for dinner tonight. I'll tell him that my cardiologist advised me not to sell the house."

Before leaving the office, she smiled and hugged me, and I knew from her demeanor that she got the message.

The Greatest Generation was written by Tom Brokaw in 1998. In it, he describes the generation that grew up in the United States during the Great Depression and went on to fight in World War II. The men and women fought not for fame but because it was the "right thing to do." I have been taking care of some of these men who have lived through the Depression, World War II, and the Korean War. This generation is also known as the GI generation. It was a unique generation whose love for our country was unconditional. They suffered but never complained. After liberating the world from tyranny, they came home and started building the nation. I will call them the Salt-of-the-Earth Generation.

The women the men married were generally poorly educated and did not work. Their lives revolved around raising children and taking care of the house. Life was simple and uncomplicated; the division of labor was well defined. Most of these women depended on men to take care of the demands imposed by the outside world.

The women lived about eight to ten years longer than the men, and without men these women were poorly prepared to cope with the complicated modern world and its problems. A woman who has lived all her life under the shadow of a decent, hardworking, and God-fearing man is ill-equipped to evaluate the hidden intentions of a new companion. Dolores was scared; she was putting herself under pressure to start a new life with Jay. A stable world became shaky and alien; she did not know how to navigate it. She trusted me to help her to make the right decision.

She came to the office for a routine follow-up and pacemaker checkup. She was complaining of difficulty in breathing, which had been getting worse to the point that she was unable to walk more than a block. Both legs were swollen, and she was finding it hard to carry on a conversation like we had the last time I saw her in the office. She was unable to sleep flat and had been using pillows to prop up her head to breathe better. She had been complaining of having transient episodes of butterflies in her chest. About six weeks ago, she had a queasy feeling in the pit of her stomach that she thought was due to indigestion. She did not seek medical help, and when her daughter visited her, she was shocked to see her in this condition and persuaded her to see me.

The physical findings showed a narrow pulse pressure and a harsh hollow systolic murmur at the apex and epigastric areas.

The ECG showed a pacemaker rhythm, the echocardiogram showed a poorly contracting and dilated left ventricle, estimated ejection fraction 38 percent (55–65 percent).

She was in class III–IV congestive heart failure. Patients in class III–IV stages of congestive heart failure have high mortality risks—the annual mortality rate is 60 percent. She was very sick and needed urgent care in the hospital.

"Dolores, I am really surprised that you did not call or get help," I said.

"I am done living," she mumbled.

She was not only suffering from congestive heart failure but also from major depression. An illness can cause depression, but in her case, it was more than that. She kept on looking at the floor, fearing that making eye contact would reveal the secrets of her pain and anguish.

"Dolores, I have to admit you in the hospital to treat the congestion in the lungs. You're suffering from congestive heart failure, which can be life threatening," I said.

She did not object. She requested her daughter to take her to the hospital.

The cocktail of medications commonly used for congestive heart failure did wonders, and her response to treatment was miraculous; the difficulty in breathing improved, and she was able to sleep while lying flat without propping up her head with pillows. The heart scan showed a large apical and anterior wall aneurysm, indicating that she suffered a massive heart attack and survived. The ejection fraction calculated with a heart scan was much lower than the 38 percent seen on the echocardiogram. This was a bad prognostic sign. The odds of her living more than a year were less than 40 percent. The heart condition was more serious than I expected.

I went to see her in the hospital. She was sitting with her daughter and going over the insurance forms and the bills to be paid. She was breathing without difficulty; the color of her skin looked normal.

"How do you feel?" I asked.

"Better." She looked at me and gave me a gentle smile.

"Dolores, the tests showed that you suffered a heart attack, and it damaged the heart muscle and the valves," I explained.

"How bad?" her daughter asked.

"The heart is damaged to a point where she will need cardiac catheterization to find out whether we can correct some of the damage with heart and valve surgery; she will also need a special kind of pacemaker called an AICD to prevent the life-threatening arrhythmias. These are invasive treatment options, or I can take care of this with medicines. Let me ask your mom how she feels about it," I said.

"No heart surgery, no new pacemaker. I want you to take care of me with medicines," Dolores decided. Her daughter tried to intervene, but she signaled her to back off.

The next day, the head nurse left a message on my cell phone saying that Dolores wanted to talk to me, and she'd very much appreciate it if I examine her without the presence of residents and medical students.

"Dolores has been waiting. I hope you got the message that she wants to talk to you alone," the head nurse said when I entered the CCU.

"Yes, I got the message. Please let the resident know that I will be seeing her alone," I said.

She was sitting calmly, reading the newspaper, betraying no signs of the conflicting emotions that were brewing inside. The calmness on her face was deceptive, much like a long-dormant volcano.

"I was in this room eight years back when you saved my life by giving me the pacemaker," she said.

"Dolores, you have a good memory," I sincerely complimented her.

"There are some incidents that are difficult to forget. The memory of them is seared into the brain. In this room, we talked about the painful experiences I had while working as a nurse. I thought that was the end of my humiliation as a woman, but I was wrong. I think God has not done with me yet," she said.

She looked at me, dabbed her tears, and thanked me for listening.

"What happened with Jay?" I asked her. She was surprised that I knew what was on her mind.

After a moment of silence, she said, "I told Jay that Dr. Kumar advised me not to sell the house, and if he wanted to take this relationship to the next level, then he should sell his house and move into my house. It was too soon and might be for the wrong reasons to sell the house."

"How did he react?" I asked.

"He did not like this, especially my saying that it was too soon and for the wrong reasons. I was afraid but not desperate to be alone; I did not panic and told him what was on my mind. I did not try to make the situation any different from what it was. Since my husband died, I have learned how to relax in my quiet house, and in this situation, everything was not under my control. Splitting from Jay would be awful, but I would survive," she said.

"What happened? Was it over?" I asked.

"No, he called after a week and wanted me to know that he was not mad. He respected my decision and was sorry that he'd asked me to take this big step so soon, and most importantly, he realized that relationships are built on trust, and with love and compassion he would earn it. He invited me to go with him to Atlantic City.

"Since the death of my husband, I have not gone to Atlantic City, so I took the plunge and agreed to it. It was one of the most terrible, unpleasant, and shameful experiences I have ever had in my life," she said.

"What happened?" I asked.

"We went to a casino and played the slot machines. He had a couple of drinks at the bar and started an argument by insisting that I tell him how much money Walter left me. I told him this was not the time or the place to discuss this matter, and I would like to pay my share of the expenses. I was furious and ashamed of myself that I was sitting with this man who asked me out for the date and wanted to know how much money I had in the bank. We checked into the hotel room, which felt like a prison cell because my mind was not there. I wanted to get home once the night was over. I was surprised to see that after his suitcase was unpacked, he showed me a kinky sex magazine with photographs of couples in weird sexual situations. He wanted me to ape those acts. It was a disgusting and nauseating moment that unleashed pent-up resentment that was long brewing, and I exploded. I called him a dirty old man and warned him not to touch me. Otherwise, I would call the police. He did not understand the resentment and thought my behavior was pathological. After some time when my anger subsided, I let him touch and hug me, and we agreed to sleep like a normal man and woman.

"When I woke up in the morning, Jay was missing from the room. I thought that he must have gone to get the coffee, but I was terribly wrong. After waiting for some time, I went out looking for him, but there was no sign of him in the lobby of the hotel or the coffee shops on the boardwalk. I was worried and exhausted not knowing what had happened to him.

"After this fruitless search, I decided to go back to the hotel to inform the reception desk about my predicament and see if they could help me to find him. The receptionist at the desk said that he checked out at seven in the morning and left a message for me, whereupon he handed me an envelope.

Dolores,
   When you get up in the morning, I will be gone. This is the punishment for not doing what you were asked to do last night. You are a big girl, and I am sure coming home alone will not be difficult.
   Good-bye.
   Jay

"Realizing that he had left me stranded, I was shocked, humiliated, and scared. I didn't know how to get home. When my husband was alive, I used to go to Atlantic City with him, and he would bring me home. I had never been to Atlantic City alone, even when I was young, and now I'm at this age with poor health, a pacemaker, and arthritis in both knees. I was stuck there and did not know what to do. I was too embarrassed to call my daughter," Dolores said.

I was shocked. "How did you manage to come home?" I asked.

"After this soul-wrecking trauma and humiliation, a part of me died that morning. The hotel receptionist arranged a taxi to take me to the bus stop. I came home physically, but a part of me was crushed forever. I wake up with nightmares, sleep-walking in the house, crying and searching for my vanished half. These nightmares end when I find my vanished half in the mirror, staring at me with tears of happiness and painful resolution," she said.

Dolores did not look at me, fearing that her face would betray her; however, I knew her will to live was gone.

You could hear a pin drop in the room—as if time had interrupted its predestined journey and stopped. I was sitting next to her not knowing what to say, or how to console her. The emotional barrier between patient and doctor, which I had maintained for many years, crumbled like a sand castle. I reached out to her and squeezed her hand. She looked at me and closed her eyes, giving the message that the time had come to say the last good-bye.

Dolores complained of severe retrosternal chest pressure that had awakened her from sleep. She became diaphoretic[39] and her heart rhythm changed, starting with premature ventricular contractions and then life-threatening arrhythmias called ventricular tachycardia/fibrillation.[40] She was treated with direct current (DC) cardioversion (defibrillation),[41] followed by an infusion of antiarrhythmic amiodarone.[42] The blood test showed that she suffered a second heart attack. The additional damage to the myocardium resulted in intractable congestive heart failure (class IV congestive heart failure). She was symptomatic at rest, and minor activities such as washing up or brushing her teeth caused a worsening of symptoms.

Even after several weeks of aggressive treatment, there was no improvement. Her heart failure continued to accelerate, and her cardiac output dropped further to a dangerously low level. She was unable to carry on a long conversation as we had many times before. During routine examinations, Dolores answered most of my questions with either a yes or no because she wanted to save as much energy as possible to continue to breathe. Her reactions to this terrible sickness were remarkably calm and dignified. I did not see panic or conflict on her face.

Studies have shown that human reactions to death are complex, multifaceted, and dynamic. People tend to develop personal meanings of death, and those meanings can accordingly be negative or positive. If they are positive, then the consequences of these meanings can be comforting to those individuals.

A person who has lived a meaningful, clean, and God-defined purposeful life will never fear death. For that person, life is not the whole journey but only half of it. After death, the journey will continue.

The famous German philosopher Martin Heidegger wrote the following:

Death is inevitable for every human being, while on the other hand, it unmasks its indeterminate nature via the truth that one never knows when and how death is going to come. All human existence is embedded in time past, present and future and when considering the future, we encounter the notion of death. This then creates angst. Angst can create a clear understanding in one that death is a possible mode of existence.

Dolores's heart failure was preterminal, and she did not have much time left to live. She wanted to die peacefully. The CCU room with its monitors and other high-tech gadgets beeping was the last place she wanted to be. She wanted to spend her last days in prayer and reflection. She remembered what her teacher at nursing school used to say: "After prison, the hospital is the most stressful place to spend the last days of one's life."

After consulting with social service personnel, I decided to discharge her with home hospice care. Hospice focuses on the palliation of a terminally ill patient's pain and symptoms, and attending to their emotional and spiritual needs. Home hospice provides care to those patients who want to spend their last days of life in their own home.

The principles of modern hospice services were pioneered in the 1950s by Dame Cicely Saunders. The modern hospice movement was built on the foundation of true unconditional love and compassion for terminally ill patients.

Saunders was a registered nurse who, in 1948, fell in love with her patient, David Tasma. He was a Polish Jewish refugee who worked as a waiter after escaping from the Warsaw ghetto. He was dying of cancer.

The German program for Polish Jews was one of concentration, isolation, and eventual annihilation. The Germans isolated them from Polish society by forcing them into sealed ghettos—walled-off cities within cities—where they had to endure appalling living conditions.

That Tasma survived and escaped was a miracle he never forgot. The subhuman conditions and tremendous suffering in the hands of Nazis could not destroy the kindness and compassion for humanity that was in his heart. When he died, he bequeathed Saunders all his savings—£500 (equivalent to £13,106 in 2013)—"to be a window in your home." Tasma, a poor Polish Jew, wanted his girlfriend to build a house for the dying. This donation helped germinate the idea that would become St. Christopher's Hospice, the world's first purpose-built hospice.

Saunders claimed that after many years of thinking and planning, she sought financial help after reading Psalm 37:5: "Commit thy way unto the Lord; trust also in him; and he shall bring it to pass." St. Christopher's Hospice opened in London in 1967, and thus began the modern hospice movement.

Dolores's birthday was the day before her discharge from the hospital. She wanted to celebrate it in the hospital in the company of CCU nursing staff. She knew that this was a unique day, so she wanted to celebrate two events—the beginning and the end. She accepted her mortality and was at peace with herself.

"My grandmother used to say, 'Forgive those who trespass against you.' I had a good life with my husband—that is all that matters. Jay misbehaved, but I forgave him. I don't want to die as a bitter person," she said.

The nurses brought the cake in her room, and we celebrated her birthday. I selected a poem for this special event and requested that the head nurse recite it to her:

The Gardener LXI: Peace, My Heart

Peace my heart, let the time for
the parting be sweet.
Let it not be death but completeness.
Let love meet in memory and pain
into songs.
Let the flight through the sky end
in the folding of the wings over the
nest.
Let the last touch of your hands be
gentle like the flower of the night.
Stand still, O Beautiful End, for a
moment, and say your last words in
silence.
I bow to you and hold up my lamp
to light you on your way.

—RABINDRANATH TAGORE

She looked up and asked me to come to her, and she whispered in my ear, "Thank God I did not sell my house as Jay wanted me to. I will die in my house—the house that Walter bought and gave to me as a Mother's Day present."

She died peacefully with dignity one week after her discharge from the hospital.

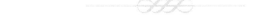

MY HEART, MY WIFE: THE STORY
OF A TOXIC MARRIAGE

"Dr. Kumar, stat to ER. Dr. Kumar, stat to ER. Dr. Kumar, stat to ER."

This was the call I received while in the middle of making teaching rounds with the medical residents at St. Peter's University Hospital. I had just finished discussing last night's admissions and helping the residents to tie up the loose ends for further workup and treatment.

"This is Dr. Kumar," I said as I called the ER.

The secretary connected me to Dr. Paul, who is head of the ER department. He and I had been working at St. Peter's University Hospital for a number of years. He was a soft-spoken, handsome, middle-aged man with blond hair and blue eyes. I had never seen him get angry or excited, despite all the problems he had to deal with in the ER.

I asked him, "What is the secret to your calmness?" He said that being vegetarian and not eating red meat keeps him peaceful and happy.

St. Peter's University Hospital is right in the heart of New Brunswick, New Jersey, home to Rutgers University and not far from Princeton University. New Brunswick is a beautiful midsize town, located about thirty-seven miles southwest of Manhattan and on the southern bank of the Raritan River. It is also known as the "Healthcare City." The corporate offices of Johnson & Johnson and Bristol-Myers Squibb are within city limits.

The city has a long and colorful history. It was given the name New Brunswick after the city of Braunschweig, Germany. It was home to Lenape Native American Indians before European settlement.

St. Peter's University Hospital is a Roman Catholic institution that opened in 1907 on Somerset and Hardenburgh Streets and moved to its present location on Easton Avenue in 1927.

When the ER called me stat, I was in the Coronary Care Unit (CCU) with the residents. In my view, the CCU is one of the best units in the hospital. The unit is not very big, and from the cardiac monitoring desk, the nurse can watch the patients as well as their cardiac monitors. The patients can sleep in peace knowing that someone is watching the monitors all the time. From the glass wall of the unit, one can see the busy traffic on Easton Avenue. Diagonally from the CCU unit is beautiful Buccleuch Park. While recuperating from a heart attack, patients can enjoy views of the park from their windows. At the entrance of the park, there is a large, majestic, and all-powerful American flag fluttering in the wind, and on the distant horizon one can see the hills of Bridgewater. The panoramic view from the CCU is the best gift St. Peter's has given to the sickest patients.

Dr. Paul said, "I have a white male who's had a massive heart attack." He gave me a brief summary of the situation.

I asked, "How old is the patient?"

"Sixty years old."

"What is his blood pressure?"

"The patient has low blood pressure, and the heart rate is very low. We are having a hard time stabilizing his blood pressure and heart rate."

I, along with the residents and medical students, interrupted our teaching rounds and rushed to the ER to the patient's room. The nursing staff was frantically working to start intravenous (IV) fluid and putting on cardiac monitor leads. Dr. Paul was, as usual, calm in directing the staff.

I introduced myself to the patient. Along with the residents, we took over the care of the patient and relieved Dr. Paul to take care of other patients in the ER.

Sal was his name, and he was a salesman for a hardware company.

"When did the chest pain start?" I asked.

"In the early morning. I thought I was having indigestion. I took an antacid, but it didn't help."

"How do you feel now?"

"I feel terrible. I'm having a hard time breathing. It feels like an elephant is sitting on my chest."

Sal was of medium height and slightly obese. His face told me the story of his life. It appeared that all his life he had been struggling to make a living. He was diaphoretic and pale. A shot of morphine had not relieved the chest pain. His blood pressure was dangerously low. He was frightened and extremely tired. I knew that if we did not move quickly, we would lose him.

"You have to save me," he said. "I don't want to die."

"We're here to help you get well. I don't want you to give up," I said.

I held his hand. That comforted him. The most important act of a doctor while taking care of a sick patient is to establish a human bond. Holding or keeping a hand on a patient's forehead for a second will do more good than we can imagine.

Sal's chest pain and breathing difficulty had not improved. We gave him an extra dose of morphine and more IV fluid. The blood pressure and heart rate stayed where they were at the time of his admission to the ER. The electrocardiogram showed that he suffered a massive inferior wall myocardial infarction.

My resident started arranging for a streptokinase infusion.[43]

Carol, our ER acute care nurse, started hooking up Sal with an external pacemaker.

The intern started working to start an extra IV line to pump more fluids to keep the blood pressure stable.

You could hear a pin drop in the room. The only sound was the low beeping coming from the cardiac monitor. Sal was lucky to reach the hospital and get help. More than 50 percent of patients die from a heart attack without getting medical attention. Most patients ignore their symptoms before the attack. There are many reasons why people do not seek help sooner. There is a strong element of the "denial factor."

It is difficult to accept the fact that we have a serious illness that can kill us. We downplay our symptoms and treat ourselves with antacids and other home remedies. The most critical factor that determines life or death is that window of time.

The window of time is about four to six hours after a heart attack. The damage to the heart muscle is time dependent. The heart muscle can recover if the blood supply to the heart is restored within the above time frame. Taking care of a patient during a heart attack requires a highly organized and dedicated medical staff. Time is life; wasting time will have devastating consequences for the patient. The patient may survive the heart attack but will suffer from heart failure due to irreversible heart damage. The objective of our treatment is to save the patient's life and prevent long-term damage to the heart muscle and heart failure.

Getting back to Sal, the cardiac monitor beeps were coming at a faster rate. I looked at the monitor. Sal's heart rate had stabilized. The medical staff taking care of Sal had been assigned specific tasks. The intern's duty was to monitor IV infusion, and the resident was monitoring streptokinase infusion. The nurse was monitoring the cardiac monitor, and Carol was assigned to manage the resuscitation cart.

"Defibrillator?"

"Charged."

"Temporary pacemaker leads?"

"Applied."

"Streptokinase infusion?"

"Running."

"IV solution?"

"Running."

Our checklist was complete.

I looked at Sal. His breathing had improved. The shining drops of sweat on his forehead had dried up. The chest pain had eased up slightly. The effect of the morphine and diazepam had relieved the anxiety on his face.

Sal looked at me, and I could see that there was a glimmer of hope in those pleading blue eyes.

Sal shut his eyes as if he were thanking me for taking care of him. I held Sal's hand and pressed it gently to let him know that I would do my best to get him out of this situation.

We had put in place a treatment plan for opening the occluded heart artery.

Clot busters are extremely dangerous drugs. There are numerous side effects, such as bleeding in the brain or the stomach that can kill the patient. There is no way of knowing how the patient will react to the medicine. The clot-buster drug acts by dissolving the clot, but when we give this drug in the IV, it will go to all the organs. If the patient has an aneurysm in the brain or a polyp in the colon, it will cause major bleeding and will kill the patient. The patient may survive the heart attack but can die from bleeding complications.

The decision to give a patient the clot-busting drug and then wait for it to work without bleeding complications is the most nerve-racking experience I go through. It is like moving slowly through a dark tunnel and praying to God to show you a ray of sunlight.

"PVCs?" the nurse at the cardiac monitor alerted me.

"Nonsustained ventricular tachycardia." Sal's heart rhythm was getting irregular.

"Defibrillator?"

"Charged and ready."

"Ventricular fibrillation?"

"Cardiovert with four hundred J. shock."

"Shocked."

"Normal sinus rhythm."

The unexpected electric shock made him jump like a fish out of water. He looked at me a bit confused and wondering what happened. This was an expected response. I'd had no time to inform him. Thank God he was heavily sedated with morphine and Versed.

When the clot-buster drug starts working, there is restoration of circulation to the heart. This will cause what we call reperfusion arrhythmia, which has to be treated within minutes. It is a life-threatening condition that, if not treated properly within minutes, will cause irreversible damage to the brain.

His reaction was a welcome sign; it gave me hope that we were moving in the right direction. It was the ray of light I was looking for in the dark tunnel.

"Normal sinus rhythm."

"EKG changes?"

"Normalized."

"Blood pressure?"

"Normal."

It took us three agonizing hours to stabilize Sal's heart attack. I looked at my residents and nurses and saw a sense of pride and accomplishment on their faces.

"There were no signs of bleeding complications from the clot-buster drug," I said.

"Thank God," Carol said. A devout Catholic, Carol always brought an element of spirituality and never forgot God. "Dr. Kumar, we are all blessed," she said.

"What do you mean?" I asked.

"There are thousands of doctors and nurses in the country, but God chose us to do his work," she said.

The faint smile on Sal's face told me that he was feeling better. He was listening to our conversation about God and his blessings. When a patient goes through a near-death experience, there is a profound change in his or her psyche. The religious differences become less important. The patient starts believing in a universal God and needs his blessing to get well. It does not matter whether the messenger is a Catholic nurse or a rabbi.

The patient's views about religion change after a major life-threatening event. It is like standing on the shore and watching the waves. There are different kinds of waves; there are big waves and small waves. The sun may be shining on some waves, and they are a pleasure to watch. Other waves are small and dark. The waves may think they are different, but the person who is watching them from the shore knows that all these waves originate from the "same ocean," and they will go back to the "same ocean." There is only "one source" where we all come from—and where we are going to go back. This is the fundamental teaching of all religions. The patient who has gone through a major illness realizes this is the true nature of God, and the man-made religious differences become less important.

There was a knock at the door. Carol opened the door and saw the ER secretary. She introduced Sal's wife who was anxious to see her husband. Carol looked at me questioningly.

"She can see her husband," I told Carol.

I looked at the woman who was standing outside the room. A slightly heavyset woman, she looked much younger than her husband. She had a round face with deep-set hazel eyes, prominent cheekbones, and a slightly protruding jaw. She was well groomed with short bobbed hair. She was wearing dark blue slacks with a beige jacket and deep-red lipstick with lots of mascara. I briefly introduced myself and assured her that her husband would be fine.

She ignored my comments and entered the room.

"Sal, goddamn it, you ruined my vacation again with this stupid heart attack," she said.

The smile on Sal's face was replaced with pain and a deep hurt. "I had no control over this heart attack. I did not plan it," he said.

"I don't care. I'm going on with my vacation as planned. I'll see you when I get back."

I told her, "This is not the time or place to talk about vacations. Sal had a major heart attack, and he almost died."

"He's done this before. Last time, I had to cancel the vacation because he was admitted to the hospital with renal colic," she said.

I looked at her with disbelief and started wondering what would happen to Sal when he was discharged from the hospital.

"You shouldn't worry about vacation. When Sal gets well, there will be plenty of time to go on vacation."

"No, it will happen again."

I could not believe that this woman, after knowing that her husband almost died from a heart attack, was still carrying on about her missed vacation. What kind of marriage was this?

"Please have a seat. Can I get you a glass of water?" Carol asked.

"No."

I looked at her face. Her tears, mixed with her mascara, trickled from her eyes down over her prominent cheekbones. Black tears meeting the red lips suddenly transformed a beautiful woman into a heartless and cruel person. She left the room, slamming the door shut.

It was my first and only encounter with her.

There was complete silence in the room. I saw anger and disbelief on Sal's face.

We all left and huddled in a conference room to discuss the further management of his heart attack.

"What about his wife's visits?" the intern asked.

I replied that she is not allowed to visit him until I have a meeting with her.

"Thank God he was sedated. Otherwise, his wife would have given him another heart attack," Carol said.

Carol wished him a speedy recovery and gave him a gentle hug, and we transferred Sal to CCU.

Next morning, his heart rate and blood pressure normalized. The electrocardiogram showed no evidence of residual heart damage.

"Dr. Kumar! Sal wants to talk to you alone," Cathy, the CCU head nurse, informed me as I entered the unit to take morning rounds.

"Good morning, Sal. How do you feel? Any more chest pain?" I found him sitting on the bed looking down, dejected, and hurt. He was beaten up both physically by the heart attack and emotionally by his wife.

"No chest pain, but I am ashamed of my wife's behavior in the ER."

"Sal, I want you to concentrate on getting well. We will talk about your wife when you see me in the office."

He stayed in the hospital for one week; his wife did not come to see him. He was discharged from the hospital and was instructed to see me in the office for follow-up.

He came to the office. He had lost weight and appeared to be under a lot of stress. Understandably, he was not over his experience in the hospital. I asked him about his health and he replied, "Physically, I'm fine."

The electrocardiogram did not show residual damage. There was no damage to the heart muscle. The clot-busting medicine did wonders for his heart. He was cured of his heart attack, but I knew that Sal would need my help to heal. My job was not done; we had a long way to go.

Next time when he came to the office, he was having a hard time making eye contact. He was quiet for some time, not knowing where to start. He was still reluctant to discuss his personal life and open his heart to a stranger. This was our second meeting out of the hospital, and I hoped this was the beginning of the healing process. I had earned his respect, but to earn his trust,

I had to talk to him man to man. My job would be to get to his core and understand his psyche and to help him heal.

Is it ethical for a doctor to get involved in a patient's personal life? I asked myself this question.

I do not know the right answer, but I know this: having gone through the fire with him and helping him beat death had created a special bond between us. His healing would take precedence over any other ethical considerations.

Finally, when he looked at me, I could see the sadness in his eyes. The trauma he suffered from his wife's behavior was still on his mind. He was having a hard time understanding and analyzing it.

He built his life around her, but instead of getting a helping hand at the time of crisis, he got a slap across his face.

"What do you think of my wife?" he asked.

"You have to tell me a little more about your marriage," I answered.

"We have been married for the last thirty years. We have no children. In the beginning of our marriage, she was remarkably supportive of my work. We had little money, but we were happy. Money is the root cause of all this trouble; it has destroyed our marriage."

"What do you mean?" I asked.

"She had an uncle who owned a travel agency. He died from a heart attack, and my wife inherited the business. Since then, our marriage has been going downhill. I am surprised to see how my wife is constantly looking for excitement. Before the money came into her life, she was a kind and considerate person. You cannot imagine how our marriage changed once my wife became economically independent."

"People change; relationships change," I said.

"What happened to this wonderful institution of marriage? What happened to the sacred vow of marriage, 'till death do us part'? I spent all my life building this relationship and see what happened?" Sal said.

"All relationships are illusions. There is nothing tangible about them. The passage of time unmasks these illusions, and then we become unhappy. The major source of our unhappiness is the belief that things will stay the same, but in reality, everything changes with time," I said.

"What about getting old? I think that age has affected my wife more than me. She is more aggressive and totally oblivious of other people's feelings. No compassion, no consideration. Her cold-blooded attitude is killing me," he said.

I was surprised to hear this. His observation about the effect of age on his wife was very close to my own.

I have been in solo private practice for the last twenty-eight years and have been taking care of couples with heart problems. I see them every three months for follow-up. The dynamics of their relationships change with time. Encroaching old age humbles a man more than a woman: he is more aware of his limitations; the lifelong struggle to raise a family has taken its toll; and the fire to fight and be a decision maker is no longer burning bright.

In the beginning of their relationship as husband and wife, the man has a slight advantage over the woman because of economics; as long as he is making more money than his wife, the relationship stays in his favor. However, once this economic advantage disappears, the relationship starts changing. A woman is not genetically programmed to support a man.

It is also difficult for a man to accept the fact that his wife is supporting him. The illusion of being in a loving and romantic marriage disappears once the economics of marriage changes. Economic independence empowers a woman and gives her a special kind of freedom. Sometimes, this newly acquired freedom can have catastrophic consequences if not used judiciously.

"What about our physical relationship?" He was too modest to say the word *sex*.

The physical relationship is important, and as we get old, the desire and performance both diminish. But, regretfully, I think money is more important in keeping a marriage going than sex.

Beep. Beep. The intercom sound distracted me from this conversation.

"Yes, Helene," I answered.

There were patients waiting to be seen. Helene knew that sometimes I got carried away with these nonmedical discussions, and that created big problems for her. Patients complained to her, and she was forced to make all kinds of excuses to defend me.

"Sal, I'd like to see you back in four weeks, and we'll continue this discussion," I said.

He came back after a week, complaining of more-frequent episodes of chest pain; plus, he had been feeling butterflies in his chest. The EKG showed no evidence of myocardial ischemia or cardiac arrhythmia.

"How does my EKG look? Am I having another heart attack?" he asked.

"No, Sal. The EKG has not changed from the last EKG, but I am worried about your complaint of feeling butterflies in your chest," I said.

"I'm never going to get well. You know what my wife said to me last night?"

"What?"

"That I am holding her back. She wants to fly, but my heart attack has clipped her wings. I feel guilty and sometimes ashamed of myself. She thinks talking to a marriage counselor is a waste of time."

"Emotional stress is one of the major risk factors for heart attack, and if you're not able to resolve this ongoing conflict with your wife, I am afraid that you will end up with another heart attack," I said.

"What should I do?" he asked. I can feel the desperation and helplessness in his voice.

"Sal, I have to think about it before I answer," I said. I was moved and touched by his trust in me. We had developed this bond where I was more than a cardiologist to him. I dreaded this responsibility of deciding about his personal life. I had no choice. He was my patient, and protecting him was part of my covenant with God. I had helped him to beat death once. I had to help him again to get this stress out of his life. Otherwise, he would end up with another heart attack and may not survive.

After Sal left my office, his problem was still on my mind. How should I guide him?

I was very much aware of my own limitations. I am trained to take care of cardiac problems, not social or marital problems. However, in his case, the marital conflicts were hindering his recovery, thus making my job more difficult. Social stress is one of the major risk factors for a heart attack. Other major risk factors are high cholesterol and smoking.

There are many drugs that can help the patient overcome stress, but these drugs have terrible side effects. For example, they can cause irregular heartbeats. The most important side effect that is painful to watch is the effect of drugs on a patient's personality. These drugs take away the pleasures of living from a patient's life. The fun of living and enjoying God's blessings is no more a part of his or her life. I do my best not to start my patients on these mind-altering drugs. I spend more time preaching than prescribing.

There are three major factors that will help the patient to beat depression and stress after a life-threatening illness: faith, family, and friends. At the time of crisis, these three Fs will help the patient to heal more than any medication I know.

To collect ashes—the charred remnants of a crisis in life—it is our faith that gives us strength and helps us to keep our sanity. Living your life without faith is like being on a rudderless ship in the ocean. In life, relationships change with the passage of time; family and friends change, but faith is like a lighthouse. It will be there in good times and bad.

In Sal's life, unfortunately, these three Fs were missing; there were no anchors to hold on to.

I was aware of this fact: my getting involved in his personal life gave him a sense of friendship and family.

Sal was readmitted to St. Peter's Hospital with chest pain. I was called to see him.

"Doc, the chest pain came back. I got scared and decided to come to the ER."

He had not suffered a heart attack. However, I admitted him for observation.

His wife never came to see him in the hospital.

I wanted to talk to his wife, but she refused to answer my calls.

"How can I live like this? This marriage isn't helping me to get well," he said. "What should I do?"

I knew the answer to his question, but I was extremely reluctant to answer him directly.

"Sal, have you heard the Sanskrit term *karmic debt?*" I asked.

"No."

"Spouses have known each other in past lives: the union between man and woman has many dimensions. You and your wife have been carrying karmic debt against each other, which has denied both of you physical, emotional, and spiritual happiness. Your suffering in this marriage is the result of past karma," I said.

Sal looked at me a bit confused. This discussion about karma was alien to him.

"I have never taken money from her. All my life I have taken care of myself; I have no debt," Sal said.

That was the end of our discussion.

It is advisable not to solve real-life problems with metaphysical remedies.

"Sal, when sociologists studied marriage and divorce, they found that people who had been in poor-quality marriages were better off getting a divorce. Divorce can be associated with improved mental health and happiness," I said.

Sal smiled. It was refreshing to see him smiling! I saw calmness on his face, the kind of calmness you see when a painful journey ends.

"Dr. Kumar, thanks very much for helping me and holding my hand. I divorced her last week."

Since then, I have lost touch with Sal. He was supposed to see me in the office, but he never called. I got a letter from him asking me to transfer his medical records. He moved out of New Jersey to a small town in Ohio.

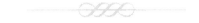

THE HISTORY AND
EVOLUTION OF MARRIAGE

Since the beginning of the twenty-first century, major social changes have led to changes in the demographics of marriage. For example, fewer people are getting married. In Europe from 1975 to 2005, there were 30 percent fewer marriages.

Most of the stories in the previous section of this book dealt with complex interpersonal relationships between spouses. As we know, this relationship is dynamic; it goes through a specific life span. It has a beginning and an end—from acquaintance to termination. What matters in life is how it ends.

To understand how this interpersonal relationship has evolved and is still evolving, it is helpful to briefly review the history of marriage.

I am well aware of the fact that eminent scholars, family historians, and other experts have written numerous scholarly papers and books on this subject. The following is my personal view of this complicated and ever-changing subject.

The history of marriage has long and colorful roots in Eastern as well as Western civilizations. In Roman history, the husband had absolute power over his wife and children. He could sell his wife to pay his debt, or put her up as collateral to continue a game of dice. The ancient Israelites regarded women as the property of the husband or father, and she could do nothing without their consent. On the other hand, divorce was easily granted. Marriage was a family matter, not a personal one, and marriages were arranged after due diligence. The duty of a wife was limited to procreation and cooperation with her husband. The concept of love-based marriage as we know it today was alien to marriage, and its importance was not well appreciated. Marriage was seen as a fundamental social institution. In ancient Greece, women were considered inferior to men. For sexual pleasure, men turned to prostitutes. The wife's role was to bear lawful offspring.

In India, the ancient Hindu culture went one step further than other ancient cultures. Marriage was a spiritual event and was considered a lifelong social and spiritual responsibility. Unlike Western culture in which humans were witnesses to a wedding, the Hindus asked the gods to witness the marriage. The marriage was a social as well as a celestial event, after carefully calculating the movement of the planets. When the constellation of stars for man and woman were in harmony, then the marriage was allowed. The goal of marriage was to have a lifelong commitment to grow spiritually. Some Hindu rituals were not allowed without the presence of the wife. However, the men continued to practice a double standard, and men enjoyed a far greater freedom and opportunity for sexual fulfillment than women.

The rise of Christianity in Europe started changing marriage laws and customs. The church gradually started preaching the gospel of sexual abstinence, and the old marriage laws were considered barbarian and un-Christian.

German laws allowed marriage to be treated as a business deal between the bridegroom and the bride's father. This was called a sale marriage. The down payment and symbol of a successful bride sale was the ring, which was given to the bride. By accepting the ring, the bride was obligated to marry the man; full payment was made at the time of the wedding. The symbolic ring ceremonies have not changed in these modern times.

The church was adamantly opposed to these barbarian laws in which the bride had no say in deciding her fate and was treated as a commodity rather than as a human being. For most of the population, marriage remained a practical and economic affair. The status of women in marriage improved, but still, they were considered inferior to men.

Marriage in modern Europe and America continued its evolution under the influence of Protestantism. The Protestant reformation started in the sixteenth century in Germany. Reformers like Martin Luther and John Calvin broke from the Catholic Church and started preaching less rigid Christian doctrines. Protestants share the core belief of Christianity, such as the doctrine of trinity and salvation through Jesus, but the interpretation of the Bible and the nature of God were entirely different. There is one God, and to receive his blessing, you do not need the help of the church or its priests. Your covenant with God to live a clean and spiritual life is the path to salvation. For Protestants, the message was more important than the messengers. Protestants have no headquarters comparable to the Vatican, where Catholics look for guidance.

For Protestant leaders like Martin Luther and John Calvin, marriage was a worldly affair, and it did not belong to a church or temple. The Catholic Church, in response to this challenge, reacted by confirming the old marriage doctrines and demanded that all marriages take place before a priest and two witnesses.

In 1630, the Puritans came to America about ten years after the Pilgrims. They were English Protestants. Unlike the Pilgrims, they did not break with the Church of England. Their leader, John Winthrop, followed the teachings of John Calvin and preached the doctrine of predestination. The Puritans' thinking about the "Nature of God" and the path to spiritual growth through contemplation and reflection was similar to what Hindus have been practicing in India since 5000 BCE. John Winthrop insisted on participation of all the believers in church activity. Only Christ was the head of the community. The covenant of grace and the covenant of works were the foundation of religion. The path to salvation was not through ossified rituals but in righteous behavior. Faith was the path to salvation.

The core of Calvinist doctrine was to decentralize the church government; this gave the Puritans church power to resist persecution and intimidation. The health of the community as a whole was equally important, and the Puritans, who considered marriage as a building block of a healthy community, did not like it to be treated as a sacrament. The Puritans made marriage secular in the new world.

The French Revolution began in 1789. The root cause of this conflict was the mismanagement of national finances. French society was divided into three groups, each representing a portion of the French population—the general French public, the clergy, and the nobility. The refusal of the church and the nobility to share the economic burden led to the execution of Louis XVI. And to diminish the power of the church, the National Convention introduced the compulsory civil marriage act. Eventually, marriage before some magistrate or government official became the only valid form of marriage. A religious wedding was permitted but had no legal status.

These two historical events—the Puritans coming to New England and the French Revolution—changed the natural history of marriage. The transformation of marriage from a socioreligious to a love-based romantic event will continue to evolve further.

The man and woman were equal in the eyes of the law, but women continued to suffer because they were dependent on men to survive. For some women, marriage was a cage. The breadwinner status of the man in marriage gave him more power than the woman.

The evolution and status of women in marriage started changing gradually with the industrial revolution. The shortage of labor to keep the factories humming brought women out of their homes and gave them a sense of economic independence.

Men started complaining about their role as breadwinners, and they resented living up to all the expectations of society at work and home. In fact, the division of labor in marriage was resented by both men and women. Women felt the breadwinner marriage was not the answer to personal evolution and fulfill-ment. This type of marriage was robbing them of their iden-tity; the suburbs were becoming "jails" for them. Women who were in traditional marriages and contented wanted a different life for their daughters. They wanted their daughters to be eco-nomically independent. They wanted their daughters to have a goal besides being a housewife and wanted them to postpone marriage to further their education.

The publication of *Playboy* by Hugh Hefner in 1953 advised men to enjoy sex without emotional or financial responsibili-ties. Women who wanted men to support them and their off-spring were called gold diggers.

Playboy turbocharged the evolution of marriage in a direc-tion that will have far-reaching consequences in the future. *Playboy* did tremendous damage to the institution of marriage. Men loved *Playboy*. By 1956, Hefner was selling more than one million copies a month.

The central role of marriage for spiritual growth and the well-being of children was questioned by *Playboy*. The mantra of "sex without responsibility" would lead to higher divorce rates. By 1957, the divorce rate in the United States started ris-ing. One in three American couples who married in the 1950s eventually divorced. Young men bragged about their sexual adventures without introspection and reflection.

A modern society was born. The worth of a man was judged by the number of sexual encounters, and walking away from women after pregnancy without shame, guilt, or respon-sibility was considered normal behavior. (Today, women brag similarly.)

For young men, Hefner was a true revolutionary, a hero who encouraged men to explore their sexuality without emotional baggage. The irony is that the Puritan Christians' way of living by the covenant of faith and reflection would be compromised by sons whose parents were Puritan Christians. That is, young men growing up without a solid foundation of faith and family would pay dearly once the "party" was over.

The reaction of women to *Playboy* would lead to further polarization of the sexes. The labeling of a wife who was also a mother—a gold digger—would set the stage for further liberation of women from conventional men who dominated in a breadwinner marriage.

The ancient Hindu culture preached the importance of marriage, a path to spiritual growth. For *Playboy* and its followers, marriage was the "jail of the soul," according to John Keats as noted in the 1957 book *The Crack in the Picture Window*.

Under feminism, the status of women in society and marriage would continue to improve; the history of feminism is the history of the growing power of women in the political and social fields. The goals and objectives of feminists were to fight for the equality of the sexes and to achieve such equality for women.

Feminism came in three waves—or tsunamis. (Unlike waves, tsunamis would change the social, political, and cultural landscape of marriage in the United States and Western Europe.)

First-wave feminism started in the nineteenth century. Democracy was men's game; women had no right to participate in elections and were not allowed to vote. Feminist leaders like

Elizabeth Cady Stanton and Susan B. Anthony fought to win women's suffrage, female education rights, and better working conditions.

First-wave feminism ended when women were finally granted universal suffrage in 1920 with the passage of the Nineteenth Amendment to the United States Constitution, which prohibited any citizen being denied the right to vote based on gender.

Second-wave feminism (1960–1980) was a continuation of the first wave; however, the goals and objectives of the feminist movement were different. After securing important rights to education, career, and voting, the feminists' objectives were to dismantle cultural inequalities and to redefine the role of women in society.

A perfect marriage with a home, children, and a hardworking husband was not enough; these women were looking for a sense of personal fulfillment, and marriage was a stumbling block in their personal evolution. Women wanted their own identity. The goals of second-wave feminists were to empower women through education and employment.

The publication of Betty Friedan's controversial book, *The Feminine Mystique*, in 1963 was a watershed event in the history of second-wave feminism and marriage. She advised women to find fulfillment and happiness outside their homes, to seek more in life than a nice home, husband, and children. The plight of women in a suffocating, breadwinner, men-dominated marriage was the main source of boredom.

Friedan was a psychologist. After the birth of her second child, she lost her job and reluctantly became a full-time mother and a traditional wife. This was a transforming event in her life. In spite of all the luxuries of modern living, she was bored and restless. Her unhappiness prompted her to write *The Feminine Mystique*. Her views about women's psyche were different than those of Sigmund Freud, who was born in Austria. He became the founding father of psychoanalysis. His views about the nature of women's psyche were highly controversial.

He said, in *Life and Work* by Ernest Jones, "The great question that has never been answered is the same one I haven't yet been able to answer, despite my thirty years of research and probing the feminine soul: What does a woman want?"

In a 1925 paper entitled, "The Psychical Consequences of the Anatomic Distinction between Sexes," Freud wrote, "Women oppose change, receive passively and add nothing of their own."

How wrong!

Friedan and other feminists criticized Freud. They believed that he was a man of his times, and his myopic views were dominated by women's sexual reproductive functions. He miserably failed to see and analyze female sexuality.

The evolution of marriage will continue. The Victorian views of female purity and gender segregation would change in second-wave feminism. Helen Gurley Brown, editor of *Cosmopolitan* magazine, advised women to use their sexuality to advance their career. As noted in *Marriage, a History* by Stephanie Coontz, Gurley Brown told women that marriage was "insurance for the worst years of your life. During your best years you don't need a husband." "You do need a man, of course, every step of the way, and they are often cheaper emotionally and a lot more fun by the bunch." Gurley Brown died at the age of ninety. There is divided opinion about her complicated legacy—whether or not she left the world a better place for women.

The biography of Gurley Brown is that of a Puritan. She faithfully remained married to the same man, and her life was devoted to her husband, her job, and her family. She was a Puritan who lived a life that was guided by a covenant of faith in the sanctity of marriage and a covenant of work.

She was an advocate of women's sexual freedom. Women could have it all—love, sex, and money. The institution of marriage was a social burden that a woman should not carry while progressing in her career. Her teachings of sexual freedom for women were similar to what Hefner preached to men in *Playboy*. However, unlike Gurley Brown, Hefner practiced what he preached.

The sexual power of women that Gurley Brown preached in *Cosmopolitan* was beautifully described by Japanese poet Yosano Akiko in 1911:

> *The time when mountains move has come.*
> *People may not believe my words,*
> *But mountains have only slept for a while.*
> *In the ancient days*
> *All mountains moved,*
> *Dancing with fire,*
> *Though you may not believe it.*
> *But oh, believe this,*
> *All women, who have slept,*
> *Wake now and move.*

Since the publication of *The Feminine Mystique*, the status of women has dramatically changed from gold digger to main breadwinner. According to a recent Pew study, in 40 percent of households, mothers are the sole breadwinners. Economic health is the most stabilizing factor in marriage. Women who are staying home are more prone to depression and at a higher risk of getting divorced.

The children of working mothers do fine. There is no evidence that this arrangement has a negative effect on their development. Studies have shown that children raised in a fatherless home do worse in society, proving the fundamental fact that children thrive in a stable marriage.

The status of women in marriage will further improve because of education, employment, and political factors. However, we should not ignore the genetic changes that are happening in the sex chromosomes.

There are two sex-determining X and Y chromosomes in mammals. The X chromosome was discovered in 1890 by Hermann Henking. Prior to discovery of y chromosome, it was presumed that the X chromosome determines sex. That was wrong. Sex determination is, in fact, due to the presence or absence of the Y chromosome.

The Y chromosome was discovered in 1905 by Nettie Stevens and identified as a sex-determining chromosome. Stevens named the chromosome *Y* simply to alphabetically follow on from Henking's *X*. Compared to most chromosomes, Y is rather small. It has about 78 protein –coding genes. In 2003, Oxford University Geneticist Bryan Sykes claimed that human Y chromosome was crumbling-dying. (The Science that

Reveals our Genetic Destiny, P.290, 2003) By one estimate, the human Y chromosome is shrinking at the rate of a genetic loss of 4.6 genes per million years. In one report, the genetic loss was estimated to be much lower.

Why is the Y chromosome in serious trouble?

The human Y chromosome is exposed to a high mutation rate. The Y chromosome is in the sperm and stored in the highly oxidative environment of the testes, which encourages further mutations. The Y chromosome does not have a "partner"- it is *Alone in the World* and lonely. No partner to talk to – or to get rid of harmful mutation through the process of genetic recombination. This inability of Y chromosome, not be able to get rid of harmful mutations is main reason for the scientists to speculate about its demise. Some scientists think it is too early to speculate about the future of Y chromosome because; further research has shown that the Y chromosome has a unique ability to self-repair itself through the process known as *gene conversion.* (Nature 423(6942):873-876, 2003).

The X chromosome in women is stable and is constantly improving by exchanging positive genetic material with the paired X chromosome.

Are these mutations in the Y chromosome partially responsible for the difficulties men are facing to adapt to twenty-first-century challenges?

Is the positive evolution happening in the X chromosome making women more assertive, and are they now adapting to the changing world much faster than men?

These are important questions to think about. The status of women in marriage as well as in the workforce will continue to improve regardless of how some men feel about it.

Men who made laws to discourage women from participating in the evolution of humanity are bound to fail because the changes in the X chromosome are too forceful to stop.

The tsunami is coming—just watch!

The paradigm shift that we see in modern marriage is due to social, political, and I think, genetic changes.

The moment of change has arrived where men must cross the divide and meet women halfway. The institution of marriage will continue to evolve. After experimenting with different kinds of relationships, both men and women are discovering that marriage is more than a total sum of all its dimensions.

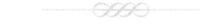

FOR MEDICAL STUDENTS

Before health management organizations (HMOs) and managed care, the physician's life was simple and uncomplicated. I started in my practice in that era. I had plenty of time to think and talk about important topics, other than relative value units (RVUs) and reimbursements. After teaching rounds, my colleagues and I would sit in the cafeteria with our students and residents and have discussions about important nonmedical issues that the students would confront in their professional lives. Our mission was to make these students more than doctors—to make them healers.

Below you will read my personal recollection of some of those general topics.

You may be thinking how lucky you are to get admitted into medical school. Luck has little to do with your admission to medical school. I believe you were predestined to be here in medical school. During your training here with us, you will learn the physical signs and symptoms of different diseases and how to cure them. This institution will teach you skills to earn a handsome income. Your journey as a *healer* will be long and hard and will continue after your graduation from medical school. You will be tested again and again on your integrity and character as a physician.

The biggest pitfall that will destroy your integrity as a physician will be greed for money. This may cloud your medical judgment, and you will end up making the wrong decision for your patients. I am not preaching poverty. Money is important. You have worked hard and deserve a comfortable life. But you have to draw a line that you will never cross, regardless of the temptations that come your way to make more money.

YOUR COVENANT WITH GOD

The day you become a healer, you make a covenant with God. The word *covenant* is used throughout scripture; however, the sad part is that we in the medical profession neglect to teach this concept to our students. Let me explain the concept of covenant as I understand it and how it applies to medicine.

According to scripture, a covenant is a sovereign-administered relationship between God and his people (in this case, you). We must understand the difference between a *contract* and a *covenant*. A *contract* is an agreement between two or more parties, especially one that is written and enforceable by law. All the parties in a contract have the option to agree or decline to participate. A *covenant* has no written or enforceable agreement. There is one party (God) who has all the power to decide. God has chosen you to be his partner in this relationship. God has done you a favor. You had no say in this covenant. The covenant relationship does not depend on the initiative of a man or woman. It is purely an act of God. God has decided to make you a partner in this relationship. The concept of a covenant in medicine is to do God's work and take care of his children. You are his partner. In short, your role as a doctor is fulfilling your end of the deal. Your actions as a doctor are accountable only to God. Once you understand the concept of the covenant, then the practice of medicine becomes a vocation rather than a business. When you are faced with difficult medical decisions and the best medical decision is being clouded by monetary gain, the covenant with God will be your guiding star. I don't know a person who has learned how to swim by reading books about swimming. You can only learn swimming by getting in a pool and practicing. You can read all about the covenant, but it has no meaning unless you apply it in your practice.

The worth of a doctor is either infinite or zero. Your compassion for and kindness to your patients will help them to heal. The practice of medicine with the covenant as your guiding principle will make you invaluable. The worth of your contribution to society is infinite. You cannot feign your compassion; it has its own vibrations and its own energy, and patients will feel that energy. With unconditional love and compassion, you will be able to establish a strong bond with your patient.

It is imperative for a doctor to establish this relationship because this bond will act as a bridge to take you to the inner core of your patient. The inner core is metaphysical. It is a combination of a person's faith in God, his or her culture, fears, and attitude toward sickness. The inner core gives meaning to a person's life. It gives him or her profound satisfaction when he or she is able to take care of the many responsibilities.

How do you understand the core of your patient? This will come through experience. This critical knowledge is part of your evolution as a physician. The most important thing is to interact and communicate with your patients on a human level. Through this genuine interaction, you will acquire a better understanding of their nature. A better understanding of your patient's nature will allow you to understand the core of your patient.

In this technological age, this may sound odd. However, no amount of technology will tell you about the core of your patient. A patient who has suffered a heart attack can be treated with a combination of medication and surgery. However, no medicine or surgical procedure can help a heart attack sufferer to overcome the emotional scar that the heart attack has left. The doctor's role is not only to treat the physical aspects of an ailment, but to heal the patient emotionally and spiritually. A doctor must understand the difference between a cure and healing. It is very easy for us to cure our patients. To heal them is not so easy. It requires your understanding of the patient's inner core.

Let us elaborate on the concept of healing. What is the difference between curing and healing? Suppose you possess something that you value the most—a piece of jewelry, a camera, and so forth. One day when you come back from work, you are surprised to find that somebody has broken into your apartment and has stolen the article most dear to you. You are hurt, angry, and miserable because someone violated your world. You want to find that person and hurt him or her. You report this to the police.

After waiting some time, you get a call from the police informing you that they have arrested the person who has stolen the article, and you are asked to collect it. When you get the precious article back, you are still mad and still hurting. The thought of somebody taking it without your permission makes you angry, and this feeling of hurt and pain may stay for some time or forever.

Let us use the same scenario for our patients. When people get sick, they feel as if somebody has taken their most valuable and precious possession (their health). They are hurt, angry, sad, and nervous. When we treat patients, we take care of the physical part of their ailments. What about the psychological trauma? When a doctor takes care of a psychological aspect of the patient's disease, then the healing starts.

Technology will help you in curing your patients, but *healing* will always come from you. Healing will come when you understand a patient's inner core. God has given you the responsibility as a doctor to heal the patient. The healing of the patient is an important component of your covenant with God.

Life is an organized instability.

What we perceive as a stable life is really an organized instability, as elaborated by David Brooks in a *New York Times* editorial. If we can understand this profound concept, then an unexpected tragedy or misfortune is easy to explain. The very nature of our existence on Earth is a state of organized instability.

Let us elaborate on this concept. Let's go to a beach and make a sand castle—a slow, step-by-step process. You keep on adding sand particles, and a point will come when you have created some sturdy-looking towers. You are not satisfied and want to make slightly higher towers. As you add more sand, the towers fall and become nothing but a pile of sand. Why? The sturdy-looking towers were an illusion. The towers looked stable from the outside, but internally they were in a state of organized instability, which was there right from the beginning when we started creating the castle.

Can we predict how much sand is needed to build a stable sand castle?

The above problem was given to IBM computer scientists. The scientists designed an experiment. They constructed the castle by adding one sand particle at a time. Then they collected all the sand particles and counted them. A special computer program analyzed the weight, size, and shape of each sand particle.

They gathered a huge amount of data from the sand particles. They believed that everything that could be measured was measured, that the data would predict the future. This assumption turned out to be wrong. The amount of sand needed to create a stable sand castle was very different each time.

Technology can do remarkable things, but predicting future events is not one of them. The computer cannot calculate the relationship between sand particles in the castle. This relationship is the foundation on which stability is dependent.

Similarly, we are not able to predict when a tragedy will strike and unravel the illusion of a stable life. As physicians, we will see patients' lives being disrupted by unexpected illness. The illusion of stability disappears with the blink of an eye. This should not surprise us. This is the way nature operates.

We live in this world where technology is replacing the human touch, which is the most important act in the care of patients. We are busy looking at the computer when our patients come to see us and collecting all kinds of useless data that have no role in the healing process. In short, the bond between a doctor and patient is being compromised. We think that with the help of technology we will transform the medical profession. The medical profession cannot be a high-tech enterprise. The bond between a patient and doctor is the foundation of our profession. This is the most sacred aspect of our existence as physicians. The patients' trust and love for you is the foundation of this bond, and if we in the medical profession let this bond die for the sake of efficiency and useless data collection, then it will be the end of our mission and calling as healers.

NOTES

1. Coronary Artery Disease—when the major blood vessels that supply oxygen and nutrients to the heart become diseased.

2. Abdominal aortic aneurysm—an enlargement of the aorta, the main blood vessel that delivers blood to the body

3. Carotid Bruit—noise caused by turbulent blood flow in the carotid arteries

4. Crepitation—a cracking sound made in breathing by a person with a diseased lung

5. Emphysema—lung disease that prevents adequate airflow and causes difficulty breathing

6. S4 gallop—abnormal heart sound

7. Murmur—sound produced when blood flows through a heart valve

8. Peripheral vascular disease—disease where narrowed blood vessels reduce blood to the limbs

9. Angina—chest pain

10. Cardiac catheterization—a medical procedure used to diagnose and treat cardiovascular conditions

11. Subtotal stenosis—severe degree of narrowing of a coronary artery

12. Revascularization—restoring necessary blood flow to the heart

13. Nocturnal dyspnea—attacks of shortness of breath that awakens the patient from sleep

14. Carotid arteries—large blood vessels in neck that supply blood to neck, face, and brain

15. RVU—measure of value used in the Medicare reimbursement formula for physician services

16. Anterolateral myocardial infarction—heart attack

17. Mitral valve insufficiency—leaking of the mitral valve

18. Tricuspid valve insufficiency—leaking of the tricuspid valve

19 Congestive Heart Failure—when the heart is unable to meet the metabolic needs of the body while maintaining normal ventricular filling pressures

20. Forward failure (low cardiac output) as well as backward failure (increased filling pressures)

21. Cardiogenic shock—heart has been damaged to the point where it cannot supply enough blood to the organs of the body

22. Pulmonary edema—excess fluid in the lungs

23. Coronary artery bypass grafts (CABG)—a form of bypass surgery that can create new routes around narrowed and blocked arteries

24. Inotropes—medications to increase the strength of the heart muscle contraction

25. Diuretics—medications that reduce the amount of salt and water in the body

26. Cardiac arrhythmia—abnormal heart rhythm

27. Ischemic cardiomyopathy—weakened and dysfunctional heart muscle often from prior coronary artery disease

28. Atherosclerotic plaque—the buildup of a waxy plaque on the inside of vessels

29. PCI—nonsurgical procedure used to treat narrowed coronary arteries

30. Angiogram—X-ray test that uses special dye to take a picture of blood flow in an artery

31. Gerontophobia—fear of growing old

32. Microembolization—a small blood clot that blocks a small artery

33. Left ventricle hypertrophy—thickened heart muscle

34. Carotid Doppler—test to evaluate blood flow velocities within the cervical carotid arteries

35. Acute infarct—heart attack

36. Monogenic genetic disorder—a medical disease caused by a DNA abnormality that can be inherited

37. Neurological defect—a problem with nerves, spinal cord, or brain

38. Thrombolytic agent—medication used to dissolve blood clots

39. Diaphoretic—sweating profusely

40. Ventricular tachycardia/ventricular fibrillation—arrhythmia that may lead to sudden cardiac death

41. Cardioversion (defibrillation)—a controlled electric shock in order to restore normal heart rhythm

42. Amiodarone—medication used to treat arrhythmias

43. Streptokinase—medication used to dissolve blood clots

Made in the USA
Middletown, DE
15 September 2016